THE HEALTH CARE MANAGER'S LEGAL GUIDE

Edited by

Charles R. McConnell, MBA, CM

Health Care Management and Human Resources Consultant
Ontario, New York

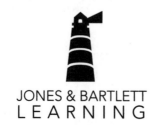

JONES & BARTLETT
LEARNING

World Headquarters

Jones & Bartlett Learning	Jones & Bartlett Learning	Jones & Bartlett Learning
40 Tall Pine Drive	Canada	International
Sudbury, MA 01776	6339 Ormindale Way	Barb House, Barb Mews
978-443-5000	Mississauga, Ontario L5V 1J2	London W6 7PA
info@jblearning.com	Canada	United Kingdom
www.jblearning.com		

Jones & Bartlett Learning books and products are available through most bookstores and online booksellers. To contact Jones & Bartlett Learning directly, call 800-832-0034, fax 978-443-8000, or visit our website, www.jblearning.com.

Substantial discounts on bulk quantities of Jones & Bartlett Learning publications are available to corporations, professional associations, and other qualified organizations. For details and specific discount information, contact the special sales department at Jones & Bartlett Learning via the above contact information or send an email to specialsales@jblearning.com.

Production Credits
Publisher: Michael Brown
Associate Editor: Catie Heverling
Editorial Assistant: Teresa Reilly
Associate Production Editor: Lisa Lamenzo
Associate Production Editor: Julia Waugaman
Senior Marketing Manager: Sophie Fleck
Manufacturing and Inventory Control Supervisor: Amy Bacus
Composition: Datastream Content Solutions, LLC/Absolute Service, Inc.
Cover Design: Kate Ternullo
Cover Image: © Chen Ping Hung/ShutterStock, Inc.
Printing and Binding: Malloy, Inc.
Cover Printing: Malloy, Inc.

Library of Congress Cataloging-in-Publication Data
McConnell, Charles R.
  The health care manager's legal guide / Charles R. McConnell, editor.
    p. cm.
  Includes bibliographical references and index.
  ISBN-13: 978-0-7637-6620-7
  ISBN-10: 0-7637-6620-8
  1. Health facilities—Law and legislation—United States. 2. Medical personnel—Legal status, laws, etc.—
United States. 3. Health facilities—Management. I. Title.
  [DNLM: 1. Health Facility Administrators—legislation & jurisprudence—United States. 2. Health Facility
Administrators—organization & administration—United States. 3. Personnel Management—legislation &
jurisprudence—United States. 4. Personnel Management—methods—United States. WX 33 AA1]
  KF3825.M39 2011
  362.11068'3—dc22

                                   2010030797

6048

Printed in the United States of America
14 13 12 11 10   10 9 8 7 6 5 4 3 2 1

Contents

Acknowledgments

A book of this sort is referred to in educational, academic, or business publishing as a *contributed volume,* meaning, as immediately evident in the indications of chapter authorship, that a number of authors were involved in its creation. Some chapters were supplied by individual authors and some by author teams of two or three. Thus, this volume includes the contributions of 20 authors, all of whom applied their various areas of expertise to provide the guidance found within these pages. The various contributors are identified with each chapter, and brief biographical entries for all are provided in the Contributors section following the About the Editor.

To the people involved in making this book possible:

- Sincere thanks to the contributing authors who took time from their busy schedules to share their expertise: Tejal P. Banker, JD, LLM; Carol A. Campbell, DBA, RHIA, FAHIMA; Ashish Chandra, MMS, MBA, PhD; Sandra K. Collins, BS, MBA, PhD; Kendall H. Cortelyou-Ward, PhD; Stephen Martin Crow, BS, MS, PhD; Susie T. Harris, PhD, MBA, RHIA, CCS; Joan M. Kiel, PhD, CHPS; Clifford M. Koen, Jr., BBA, MS, JD; Robert R. Kulesher, PhD, FACHE; Aaron Liberman, PhD, LHRM; Eric P. Matthews, PhD, RT(R)(CV)(MR); Michael S. Mitchell, JD, LLM; Dawn M. Oetjen, PhD; Reid Oetjen, PhD; Bianca Perez, MS; Llewellyn E. Piper, PhD; Timothy Rotarius, PhD, MBA, BBA; and Andrea Velez-Vazquez, BS, MS.

- Special thanks to Clifford M. Koen, Jr., and Michael S. Mitchell for their legal review of several chapters.

- Additional thanks to Clifford M. Koen, Jr., Associate Professor of Business Law at the College of Business and Technology, East Tennessee State University, who, in addition to reviewing several chapters during an especially busy period, generously shared some of his original material to expand the contents of Chapter 8.

- Thanks to the crew at Jones & Bartlett Learning for always being a pleasure to work with.

- Special thanks to Michael Brown, Publisher, who first put forth the idea for this book and with whom I have worked on numerous projects for more years than either of us may readily admit.

Charles R. McConnell
Ontario, New York

Getting the Job Done While Avoiding Legal Hassles

The above title describes the purpose of this book in a nutshell. A slightly longer statement of purpose is: *To provide guidance for the working healthcare manager who must manage day to day in an environment littered with potential legal pitfalls.* There are hazards related to recruiting, interviewing, and reference checking; wage and salary issues, including describing and grading jobs and the approval and control of overtime; maintaining patient and employee privacy and confidentiality; determining employee eligibility for various legislated benefits such as the Family and Medical Leave Act; addressing allegations of sexual harassment in particular and dealing with disciplinary matters in general; governing management behavior during union organizing; and a number of other concerns involving situations in which the manager might encounter legal issues in everyday operations.

Consider the following example: today's experienced interviewers know that it is illegal under Title VII of the Civil Rights Act of 1964 to ask a job applicant about any aspect of marital or family status. They further know that even if an applicant reveals such personal information during an interview, the interviewing manager cannot legally use this information in making a hiring decision. The case in point: a young woman applying for an entry-level technician position said directly to the interviewing manager, "I'm pregnant and if you don't hire me I'll charge discrimination." This statement was heard by no one other than the interviewer, so there were no witnesses. What was the manager to do?

The interviewing manager in question was aware that the personal information obtained could not be allowed to influence a hiring decision. The applicant's bluntly stated threat prompted the manager, following advice from knowledgeable sources in the organization, to carefully document the interview results for all candidates for the position, carefully compare the qualifications of all candidates, and prepare to defend, if necessary, the offer of the job to the apparently best-qualified applicant. The bold applicant was not hired; however, the complaint she filed with the state's Division of Human Rights was dismissed on initial investigation because the employer could demonstrate that the person hired was the best-qualified applicant.

Without solid documentation and the ability to reasonably show that the best-qualified applicant was chosen, upon turning down the threatening applicant, the manager could well have become involved in a prolonged dispute.

Legal regulation of employment essentially began in the 1930s with passage of the Fair Labor Standards Act and the National Labor Relations Act. However, it was the Civil Rights Act of 1964 that began the modern era of government regulation of employment that work organizations face today. Since 1964, there has been a series of new laws and amendments to laws, many of which have direct as well as indirect effects on managers—those employees who must oversee and guide the efforts of other employees.

Surely there are more topic areas in addition to the 15 addressed in this book that could have been included. However, for most healthcare managers, the topics covered within these pages likely address the majority of legal pitfalls they are likely to encounter. For example:

- At one time or another, nearly all managers find it necessary to select new employees, so the legal pitfalls involved in interviewing and reference checking are reviewed.

- Most managers sometimes find it necessary to discipline or even discharge an employee, so the ways to go about this less than pleasant task with minimal legal risk are offered.

- Today's focus on sexual harassment and the prevalence of charges of sexual harassment suggests the need for the manager to know what is best to do when confronted with such issues.

- Some managers direct unionized employees and many managers become exposed to union organizing, so guidance is offered for managing under such conditions while steering clear of legal obstacles.

- Managers sometimes find themselves involved in employment-related lawsuits or other legal proceedings, so guidance is presented for managers' behavior when so involved.

There is necessarily a limited amount of overlap between and among certain chapters. For example, Chapters 5 and 6 both address antidiscrimination laws to some extent, and Chapters 10, 13, and 15 all describe the legal process of *discovery*, although from somewhat differing perspectives.

The chapters in this volume have been contributed by both practitioners and educators, including several who have been or are presently both an educator and practitioner, and several who are attorneys as well.

It is essential that the reader or user of *The Health Care Manager's Legal Guide* recognize that *nothing presented in this book is intended as legal advice*. This book simply provides information and general guidance. Some of the material in these pages has been supplied by attorneys, some was supplied by knowledgeable practitioners and educators, and most has been reviewed by attorneys. Use this book to become sufficiently knowledgeable of legal pitfalls so you can do your best to avoid them; a hazard avoided is a potential problem likewise avoided. Thus the primary theme of this book is *avoidance* of legal problems. But when an unavoidable real-world legal problem arises, rely on your organization's legal counsel.

Charles R. McConnell, MBA, CM

Charles R. McConnell is an independent healthcare management and human resources consultant and freelance writer specializing in business, management, health administration, and human resource topics. For 11 years, he was a management engineering consultant and director of personnel development and training with the Management and Planning Services (MAPS) division of the Hospital Association of New York State (HANYS), and later spent 18 years as a hospital human resources manager. As author, coauthor, and anthology editor, he has published 28 books and has contributed nearly 500 articles to various publications. He is in his 29th year as editor of the quarterly professional journal, *The Health Care Manager.*

Mr. McConnell received a BS in industrial engineering and an MBA, both from the State University of New York at Buffalo, New York.

Tejal P. Banker, JD, LLM

Tejal P. Banker is a healthcare attorney who specializes in representing individual healthcare providers such as physicians, nurses, and psychologists and healthcare facilities such as imaging centers, surgery centers, hospitals, and clinical and pathology laboratories, in a variety of transactional healthcare matters. Ms. Banker's legal practice focuses on ensuring that healthcare transactions undertaken by her clients comply with state and federal healthcare fraud and abuse legislation. Ms. Banker has published numerous articles addressing healthcare fraud and abuse and has frequently lectured on this topic. In addition to practicing law, Ms. Banker serves as an adjunct faculty member in the Healthcare Administration program at the University of Houston, Clear Lake, in Houston, Texas. Ms. Banker received her juris doctorate from Southern Methodist University in Dallas, Texas, and her master's degree in healthcare law from the University of Houston in Houston, Texas.

Carol A. Campbell, DBA, RHIA, FAHIMA

Carol A. Campbell joined the Medical College of Georgia (MCG) in 1984 and is currently a professor in the Department of Health Informatics, School of Allied Health Sciences (SAHS). Dr. Campbell served as chair of the Department of Health Informatics from 1998 to 2007. From 2001 to 2009, she also served as an associate dean in the SAHS at MCG. Prior to her academic career, she served as the regional director for a health maintenance organization (HMO) in Southern California. Dr. Campbell has published and presented nationally and internationally on diverse topics including strategic planning, distance education, curriculum design and implementation, integrated practice management systems, leadership, and enlightened self-interest.

Dr. Campbell has an undergraduate degree in Medical Record Administration from Loma Linda University, a master of arts in management from the University of Redlands, and a doctorate in business administration from Nova Southeastern University. She is credentialed as a registered health information administrator (RHIA) and she is fellow of the American Health Information Management Association.

Ashish Chandra, MMS, MBA, PhD

Dr. Chandra is a professor and department chair of healthcare administration at the University of Houston, Clear Lake, in Houston, Texas. He has authored or coauthored over 50 articles for professional journals and nearly 200 conference proceedings. Active in several professional associations, he has served as the president of the Business and Health Administration Association, the Association of Collegiate Marketing Educators, the MBAA International, and the Federation of Business Disciplines. He also serves on the boards of the Asian Health Care Leaders Association and the American College of Healthcare Executives, Southeast Texas Chapter. He is currently an executive editor of *Hospital Topics* and serves on the editorial boards of several professional journals.

Dr. Chandra earned a BS (Statistics) and MMS (Marketing) from Banaras Hindu University in India, and an MBA and PhD from the University of Louisiana, Monroe. Prior to joining the University of Houston, Clear Lake, he was a faculty member and coordinator of the Graduate Healthcare Administration Program at Marshall University in West Virginia, and earlier was a faculty member at Xavier University of Louisiana in New Orleans. Dr. Chandra has received numerous teaching, research, and service awards.

Sandra K. Collins, BS, MBA, PhD

Sandra K. Collins is an associate professor in the Health Care Management Program within the School of Allied Health at Southern Illinois University, Carbondale. She has approximately 17 years experience in the management of healthcare-related facilities and has authored numerous publications concerning human resource aspects related to the healthcare field. She has also served as a state, national, and international speaker on a variety of management-related topics.

Dr. Collins received her BS, MBA, and her PhD in workforce education and development from Southern Illinois University, Carbondale.

Kendall H. Cortelyou-Ward, PhD

Kendall Cortelyou-Ward is the director of the Health Services Administration undergraduate program at the University of Central Florida. Dr. Cortelyou-Ward earned her bachelor of science degree in human resource development from the University of Florida and her master of science and PhD in health administration from the University of Central Florida. She has authored numerous peer-reviewed presentations and publications on issues of human resources in health care. Her research interests revolve around workflow processes, employee commitment, and human resource development.

Stephen Martin Crow, BS, MS, PhD

Stephen Martin Crow is the endowed chair and professor of Healthcare Management at the University of New Orleans. He is also an adjunct professor at the Louisiana State University Health Science Center, Department of Public Health. Dr. Crow has been with the University of New Orleans for over 20 years. Prior to that, he was a human resource management professional for a variety of organizations for more than 20 years. He also serves as an arbitrator with the Federal Mediation and Conciliation Services.

Dr. Crow received a BS at Louisiana State University and an MS and PhD at the University of North Texas. He resides in Covington, Louisiana, with his lovely wife Suzanne, two Airedales, two mixed breeds, and three feral cats. He is an avid motorcyclist, having toured extensively in the United States, Europe, South Africa, New Zealand, and South America. With a last name of Crow and middle name of Martin, it is only natural the he is an extensive watcher, landlord, and feeder of local birds.

Susie T. Harris, PhD, MBA, RHIA, CCS

Susie T. Harris is an assistant professor in the Department of Health Services and Information Management at East Carolina University. She received her undergraduate degree in health information management, her MBA with a concentration in healthcare administration, and doctor of philosophy degree in rehabilitation studies, all from East Carolina University. She has 17 years of experience in healthcare administration. Her areas of interest are health industry education, coding, managed health care, electronic exchange of health information, diabetes, and spirituality.

Joan M. Kiel, PhD, CHPS

Joan M. Kiel is the chairman of the University HIPAA Compliance and associate professor of Health Management Systems at Duquesne University in Pittsburgh, Pennsylvania. She is also the voluntary chairman of the American College Health Association National HIPAA/HIM Coalition. Dr. Kiel is certified in healthcare privacy and security. She has written extensively on HIPAA and health management topics as well as given international, national, and regional presentations. She received her doctorate from New York University.

Clifford M. Koen, Jr., BBA, MS, JD

Clifford M. Koen is an associate professor of business law at East Tennessee State University. For over 20 years he has taught undergraduate and graduate courses in employment law, business law, and human resource management. He has also served as a consultant and trainer on a variety of human resource topics including equal employment opportunity legislation, sexual harassment, employee discipline, performance appraisal, and employment interviewing. Prior to beginning his career in academics and consulting, he had 10 years of experience in human resource management in the healthcare and petroleum industries. He is a frequent public speaker and has authored and coauthored numerous publications for professional journals.

Robert R. Kulesher, PhD, FACHE

Robert R. Kulesher is a health policy specialist and experienced hospital and nursing home administrator. He holds a BA in psychology from Villanova University, a master of health administration from Washington University in St. Louis, and, following a 20-year career in healthcare administration, a PhD in urban affairs and public policy from the University of Delaware. His research focuses on the impact of Medicare reimbursement on healthcare providers; additional areas of interest include national health policy, healthcare financial management, health care for the poor and uninsured, health insurance, Medicare, and Medicaid. Dr. Kulesher is director of the Health Services Management program in the Department of Health Services and Information Management at East Carolina University. He previously held faculty appointments at Penn State, St. Joseph's University, and Rutgers University, Camden as visiting professor in public policy and administration.

Aaron Liberman, PhD, LHRM

Aaron Liberman currently is professor of health services administration at the University of Central Florida in Orlando and also serves as interim chairman of the department. Dr. Liberman is a qualified hospital administrator and has worked actively in the field for more than 20 years managing hospitals and health services organizations.

As a researcher, Dr. Liberman has published more than 80 scholarly manuscripts in refereed national and international journals, five monographs, and three books. He has recently completed a fourth book entitled *Raising a Parent*. He serves as a member of the editorial review board of two national journals and is a charter faculty fellow of UCF's Academy of Teaching, Learning and Leadership.

Dr. Liberman has earned four academic degrees: a bachelor of arts in psychology from Baylor University, a master of science in educational psychology from Indiana University, a master of arts in hospital and health administration from the University of Iowa, and a PhD in hospital and health administration from Iowa.

Dr. Liberman and his wife Joan S. Liberman, a licensed clinical social worker and psychotherapist in private practice, are the parents of two grown children and have three grandchildren. They reside in Orlando.

Eric P. Matthews, PhD, RT(R)(CV)(MR)

Eric P. Matthews is an assistant professor in the College of Applied Sciences and Arts, Southern Illinois University, Carbondale (SIU). He has taught within the School of Allied Health at SIU for 8 years; he also has over 18 years experience in diagnostic imaging, ranging from large trauma centers and teaching hospitals to outpatient imaging facilities. He has published a wide range of articles and given numerous presentations, both nationally and internationally, on topics ranging from 19th century medical history to modern medical ethics and law.

Michael S. Mitchell, JD, LLM

Michael S. Mitchell is a founding partner of the New Orleans office of Fisher & Phillips, LLP. His practice covers all aspects of employee relations, with an emphasis on collective bargaining, defense of unfair labor practice charges, union avoidance, and supervisor training.

Mr. Mitchell graduated from the West Virginia University College of Law in 1973 and for four years served in the judge advocate corps of the US Air Force as trial counsel. He earned a master's degree in labor law from George Washington University, magna cum laude, in 1979. He has been recognized by *The Best Lawyers in America* as one of America's leading labor and employment lawyers, as well as in *Chambers Partner* and *Who's Who in Law,* and was named by *New Orleans Magazine* as one of the best lawyers in the city. He is a member of the Global Association of Hotel Attorneys, a frequent speaker before trade and professional associations, and is the editor of the firm's award-winning newsletters, practice area publications, and legal compendiums.

Dawn M. Oetjen, PhD

Dawn M. Oetjen is an associate professor and program director for the graduate program in Health Services Administration, Department of Health Management and Informatics, College of Health and Public Affairs at the University of Central Florida. Her teaching focus has included healthcare quality management, health information management, research methods, epidemiology, and healthcare law and ethics.

Dr. Oetjen has numerous peer-reviewed publications and regularly presents her research at academic and practitioner conferences. Her research efforts focus on management, ethics, and education. She has also served as the director of quality management, case management, utilization review, health information management, and support services in acute care, rehabilitation, and mental health facilities. She received her undergraduate degree in health information management and her graduate degree in health administration from the Medical University of South Carolina and her doctorate from the University of Alabama at Birmingham.

Reid Oetjen, PhD

Reid Oetjen is an assistant professor and director of the Executive Health Services Administration (e-MSHSA) Graduate Program in the Department of Health Management and Informatics at the University of Central Florida. He teaches courses at both the undergraduate and graduate levels focusing on long-term care administration, healthcare quality management, human resources management, and the aging of the population.

Dr. Oetjen has numerous peer-reviewed publications and regularly presents his research at academic and practitioner conferences. His research foci are on the quality of long-term care, development of tools for healthcare practitioners, and the scholarship of teaching and learning. Dr. Oetjen previously served as an assistant administrator for a national skilled nursing facility chain and spent 10 years as an operations manager for a major international airline.

Bianca Perez, MS

Bianca Perez is a doctoral student at the University of Central Florida in Orlando where she is pursuing a degree in public affairs with a concentration in health services administration. She currently works for the Health Services Administration Department as a teaching and research assistant. Previously, she attended McGill University in Montreal, Canada, where she obtained a bachelor of arts in psychology, and Carlos Albizu University in Miami, where she obtained a master of science in industrial organizational psychology.

Llewellyn E. Piper, PhD

Llewellyn E. Piper is president and chief executive officer of Onslow Memorial Hospital, Jacksonville, North Carolina. He is an adjunct instructor in psychology at Campbell University where, over a period of more than 15 years, he has also taught industrial psychology, research methods, clinical psychology, perception, abnormal psychology, and other subjects. His experience in healthcare management and leadership spans nearly 40 years, including 21 years as an officer in the U.S. Army Medical Service Corps. He has published more than a dozen articles addressing such topics as management, leadership, ethics, trust, and human motivation.

Dr. Piper received a BS in biology at The Citadel and a master's degree in healthcare management at Baylor University. He holds several other master's degrees in addition to his doctorate.

Timothy Rotarius, PhD, MBA, BBA

Timothy Rotarius is a professor of health services administration and vice chair of the Department of Health Management and Informatics in the College of Health and

Public Affairs at the University of Central Florida. His research focuses on health-care finance and healthcare management and includes 65 peer-reviewed publications and 70 presentations to academic and professional associations.

Dr. Rotarius has served as program director of a 500-student BS-health services administration degree, an internship coordinator for hundreds of health services administration student internships, and a program director of a 250-student MS-health services administration degree. He earned a PhD in healthcare strategic management from Texas Tech University, which complements his MBA and BBA in finance. Dr. Rotarius has 12 years of professional experience in the financial management field, and he regularly serves as a consultant to large and small business organizations.

Andrea Velez-Vazquez, BS, MS

Andrea Velez-Vazquez is the academic coordinator of the Health Management and Informatics Department in the College of Health and Public Affairs at the University of Central Florida. She has worked in different capacities in academia focusing on the areas of developmental advising, recruitment, training, and personnel development. She has done extensive research on numerous topics in the field of human resources. Mrs. Velez-Vazquez received her BS in criminal justice from the University of Central Florida and her MS in human resources management from Nova Southeastern University.

Chapter 1

Wage and Hour Laws: Every Manager's Concern

Charles R. McConnell, BS, MBA, CM, *Healthcare Management and Human Resources Consultant, Ontario, New York*

Chapter Objectives

- Review the origins of the Fair Labor Standards Act (FLSA) and develop an understanding of the rationale for its passage.
- Focus attention on the portions of the FLSA that are pertinent to the majority of working healthcare managers.
- Address the meanings of and the differences between the employee classifications "exempt" and "nonexempt" and how these impact the healthcare manager's role.
- Address "overtime" and the problems attendant to its determination, payment, and control.
- Enumerate the manager's responsibilities relative to wage and hour legislation.

The Beginning: The Fair Labor Standards Act

The Fair Labor Standards Act (FLSA), passed into law in 1938, is the basic federal wage and hour law. Since its passage, it has been the basis of essentially all legislation affecting wages and hours in the workplace, serving as a model for the wage and hour laws of many individual states. There is considerable variation among state laws; some states are heavily reliant on the federal law while certain other states have wage and hour laws of their own, some preceding the federal law and some addressing a few unique issues that the FLSA does not address. As is always the case when the same practices are addressed by both federal and state laws, the more stringent of the two is the one that applies in any given situation. However, the FLSA is relatively comprehensive and thus in a practical sense, it negates the need for extensive detail in state legislation. Because the FLSA is more comprehensive and far-reaching than the wage and hour laws of most states, it essentially serves as the country's basic wage-and-hour legislation.

The FLSA is administered by the Wage and Hour Division of the US Department of Labor (DOL). It has been amended several times since 1938, with one of the more prominent amendments being the Equal Pay Act of 1963.

At one time in the not-too-distant past, certain healthcare organizations, specifically providers such as hospitals, were exempt from the minimum wage and overtime requirements of the FLSA. Such organizations were not required to—and some at the time did not—pay minimum wage or pay for overtime. However, amendments to the FLSA passed in 1967 required that the law's minimum wage and overtime requirements must apply equally to healthcare organizations as to organizations in other industries.

Congressional Intent

In passing the FLSA, one of the apparent objectives of the US Congress was to reduce the high unemployment rate that typified the 1930s, the decade of the Great Depression. The FLSA did so by reducing the number of hours in a workweek to a uniform standard, thus attempting to spread available work over a greater number of workers. In addition to defining a so-called normal or standard workweek, the FLSA set minimum rates of pay, established rules for the payment of overtime, and regulated the employment of minors.

The FLSA is a lengthy and detailed body of legislation that addresses many aspects of employment. Only a few parts of this legislation are immediately pertinent to the majority of healthcare department managers. Foremost among these are the portions of the law addressing employee classification, hours of work, and the payment of overtime. A few parts of the FLSA, in particular the minimum wage and child labor requirements, affect other departments within the organization. For example, in securing job candidates, the human resources department will not refer for interview any job applicants who are not of legal age to do the kind of work involved or work the number of hours or shifts required (the threshold for employment in the majority of positions in the healthcare organization is age 18). The minimum wage provisions of the FLSA are also of concern to administration, human resources, and the finance department, since some such organizations still start their unskilled entry-level employees at minimum wage.

Therefore, this chapter will focus on those portions of relevance to most working department managers who essentially need to know about the differences between and the treatment of *exempt employees* and *nonexempt employees*; the payment of overtime; and, by logical extension of management's concern, the control of overtime.

Employee Classifications

Exempt Employees

Most managers have heard the terms "exempt employee" and "nonexempt employee" all of their working lives. These labels mean, of course, that one is either exempt or not exempt from the minimum wage and overtime requirements of the FLSA. The applicability of the minimum wage condition can essentially be ignored as far as exempt employees are concerned; the conditions defining exempt (outlined as follows) preclude payment of compensation below some specified level.

Exempt employees, often referred to as "salaried," need not legally be paid overtime, but nonexempt employees, usually referred to as "hourly" employees, must by law receive overtime payment. These descriptions can get hazy under certain conditions. Although the law does not require overtime payment to them, some employees who otherwise qualify as exempt can be paid overtime at the convenience of the organization. For example, the majority of registered nurses working in staff positions receive overtime pay for hours worked in excess of the normal workweek even though they may be described as professionals under FLSA criteria. This is clearly a practical consideration, especially in light of chronic nursing shortages. How many nurses would readily work extended shifts or extra days without additional compensation?

Employees in any of the three following categories can legally be treated as exempt from the overtime requirements of the FLSA:

1. *Executives.* An executive employee must generally spend 50% or more of the time in direct management of an organization or organizational subunit such as a department. An executive employee must also direct the activities of two or more persons. The executive definition may also require that a person possess the authority to hire and fire or so recommend; possess discretionary powers rather than being assigned mostly routine work; and from workweek to workweek, spend no more than 40% of the time on non-managerial work.

2. *Administrative.* An administrative employee must spend 50% or more of the time on office or nonmanual work related in some way to policy, general business, patient care, or people in general, and must be required to exercise discretion and independent judgment when necessary. Other tests of the administrative classification may consist of assisting executive or other administrative personnel; handling special assignments with only general supervision; working in a position requiring special training, experience, or knowledge; and spending not more than 40% of the time on nonadministrative work.

3. *Professional.* Professionals in healthcare institutions (e.g., chemists, registered nurses, physical therapists, pharmacists, physicians) are so classified by virtue of spending 50% or more of the time in work that requires advanced specialized knowledge or is original or creative in nature. The definition may also require that the professional be consistently required to exercise discretion and independent judgment, be employed at intellectual and varied work, and be engaged in nonprofessional activities not more than 20% of the time.

The FLSA specifies the minimum salary that executive, administrative, and professional personnel must be paid. The single exception applies to licensed medical practitioners, interns, and residents; they are subject to no minimum salary requirements.

Controversies centering on the applicability of a particular nonexempt definition are frequently decided on the basis of the percentage of time spent on various activities. The time test applies on a workweek to workweek basis.

Nonexempt Employees

All employees who do not fall under the executive, administrative, or professional category are considered nonexempt employees. They must be paid at least the prevailing legal minimum wage for each hour worked in a workweek, and they must be paid at a rate of 1.5 times their "regular rate" for all overtime hours ("regular rate," addressed later in this chapter, is emphasized because it is not simply an employee's base rate of pay; differences in identifying its components have caused legal difficulty for some organizations).

The organization is required to keep detailed records of hours worked and wages paid. There are a few well-defined exceptions to the payment of the legal minimum wage; special regulations allow the payment of lower rates to students, learners, and apprentices. Employment of such persons is also subject to additional requirements and restrictions.

Which Classification?

The preceding paragraphs set forth, in summary fashion, the conditions that must be satisfied for a particular position to be labeled exempt. Any position that meets the requirements of executive, administrative, or professional *may* be designated exempt, and all positions not qualifying under these requirements *must* be designated nonexempt.

Being nonexempt is advantageous to the employee because overtime must be paid for all hours in excess of 40 in a week. Being exempt is seen by some as advantageous to the employee because of the usually associated higher rate of pay and often the flexibility of hours. The exempt designation is seen as advantageous to the employer because of the stability of labor cost that it affords and the ability to get additional work accomplished beyond 40 hours in a week without additional payment.

It is essential to recognize the difference between the uses of *may* and *must* in the preceding paragraph. The law clearly states that any position that does not meet the exempt criteria must be considered nonexempt and be paid overtime. However, a position that meets the exempt criteria is not legally required to be treated as purely exempt. It is true that many such positions are classified and treated as clearly exempt (e.g., healthcare administrators, department heads, accountants, engineers). It is equally true that some positions that qualify as exempt are, as previously noted, treated as nonexempt in that they receive overtime pay. This practice, essentially giving some employees the best of both the exempt and nonexempt worlds, exists out of practicality.

There is some risk involved in incorrectly classifying employees as exempt when they should in fact be nonexempt. In some organizations, certain positions have been treated as exempt simply because they were compensated at or above the minimum exempt salary requirement. However, because a position may not involve a sufficient percentage of true administrative work it may, upon audit by the DOL (or by the equivalent state agency), be ruled nonexempt. If this occurs, the organization will be required to pay imputed overtime costs for positions that have been incorrectly classified. For a position to be treated as exempt, it must meet the requirement for work content as well as that for salary.

The Difference Is More Than Academic

It is to the department manager's advantage not only to understand the difference between exempt and nonexempt but also to understand the FLSA requirements of each and to ensure that the department's employees are properly classified. Knowledge of FLSA employee classifications is also valuable in the creation or revision of job descriptions.

In many organizations, one can find improperly classified employees, and in fact it has been observed on many occasions that the FLSA is the one law having to do with employment that is most frequently violated by employers. Some violations are innocent, resulting from confusion or misinterpretation. However, some violations of wage and hour law result from employers deliberately bending regulations to save money.

There is always the chance that an organization's decision to designate any particular position as exempt may be challenged by the aforementioned DOL. An audit or investigation by DOL can be initiated in either of two ways: the DOL may decide to do a routine audit of the practices of an organization selected at random, or DOL investigators may descend upon the organization because they have received an employee complaint. The DOL investigators will not reveal whether they are there for a routine audit or because of a complaint.

A given complaint may involve almost any aspect of wage payment, but many of the more common complaints involve eligibility for overtime payment as determined by an employee's status as exempt or nonexempt. DOL investigators apply their judgment in comparing actual job duties with the FLSA definition criteria for executive, administrative, and professional employees. Consider the example presented by a particular practice that has caused many organizations to run afoul of the DOL: reclassifying higher-level secretaries (such as those in administration or in other senior secretarial positions) as salaried and thus exempt by raising their pay to an appropriate level (relative to the FLSA requirements) and giving them more responsible sounding titles. *Administrative assistant* is one such title often encountered. Doing so provides the flexibility of longer or varied hours when appropriate. Numerous organizations have made such changes in the apparent belief that the increased pay and title change were enough to justify the exempt designation. However, when the DOL applies the FLSA requirements to the jobs of such employees, these positions frequently do not measure up to the defining requirements of *administrative* personnel, especially as concerns the "exercise of discretion and judgment" and the percentage of time spent doing various kinds of work.

When such findings result from audit or investigation, the DOL will require that for each affected person, the hours worked in excess of 40 must be determined—often estimated, when specific records are not available—and that those hours must be compensated at an overtime rate. When the DOL concludes that the avoidance of overtime payment was not intentional, the organization will be ordered to pay imputed overtime retroactive for up to 2 years. If it is concluded that the organization was deliberately avoiding overtime costs, the payment of imputed overtime for 3 years past is required and there can be additional legal repercussions as well.

It is therefore in the best interests of the organization for the department manager to know the requirements of the FLSA and to provide critical input into the evaluation and classification of positions in the department.

Nonexempt employees are paid by the hour and are entitled to 1.5 times their "regular rate" for hours worked in excess of 40 in a week. Exempt—that is, salaried—employees are theoretically compensated for the week at the same level regardless of whether they work more or less than 40 hours. In practice, however, in most organizations' exempt employees ordinarily average in excess of 40 hours a week. As might be cynically expressed by a salaried employee trying to explain the essential difference between nonexempt and exempt: Nonexempt employees get time-and-a-half; exempt employees just get time and again.

Equal Pay

A section of the FLSA prohibits discrimination among employees on the basis of gender when the employees are doing equal work on jobs requiring equal skill, effort, and responsibility, and are performed under similar working conditions. In correcting unlawful differences in rates of pay, the FLSA requires that the lower rate be increased; it is not permissible to decrease the higher rate. The act does make provision, however, for unequal pay if the inequality is directly attributable to a bona fide seniority system, merit system, incentive compensation system, or any other plan calling for a differential in pay based on any factor other than sex.

Overtime Compensation

The Workweek

The FLSA defines the workweek as a fixed, recurring period of 168 hours; that is, 7 consecutive 24-hour periods. These 24-hour periods need not be calendar days, and the 7 periods together need not comprise a calendar week. For instance, work-weeks beginning and ending at midnight on Friday or midnight on Sunday are not uncommon. The workweek may be changed, and many organizations have done so to facilitate payroll accounting, but it cannot be changed in midstream; that is, it cannot be changed such a way as to avoid payment of overtime that has technically already been earned.

Time and One Half

The FLSA requires payment of 1.5 times a worker's regular rate for all overtime hours. Overtime hours are defined as hours worked in excess of:

- 40 hours in a 7-day workweek, where the ordinary 7-day workweek is used; or
- 8 hours per day *or* 80 hours per 14-day period, when the use of the 14-day period has been approved and posted.

The organization may use either or both methods for certain employees but may use only one method at a time for any specific employee group. If the so-called "8-and-80" provision is used, overtime must be paid for all hours worked in excess of 8 in each day or in excess of 80 in the 14-day period, whichever results in the greater number of overtime hours.

In the example shown in Exhibit 1-1, the employee worked a total of just 80 hours. However, the employee is owed 3 hours of overtime, this being derived from the 4th day, when 10 hours were worked, and the 8th day when 9 hours were worked (even though on 1 day the employee worked only 5 hours).

Consider next the situation presented in Exhibit 1-2. In this case, the employee worked more than 8 hours on 1 or more days and more than 80 hours for the 14-day period. This example assumes that the employee worked 8 hours in each of 9 days and 10 hours on the 10th day and thus is due 2 hours of overtime. Note that the employee has worked 2 hours in excess of both the 8 hours per day and 80 hours per work period provisions. However, this does not mean that the employee is entitled to overtime for 4 hours (based on 2 hours in excess of 8 and 2 hours in excess of 80). The employee is owed just 2 hours of overtime pay. Hours cannot be double-

Exhibit 1-1

"8 and 80" Example 1

Day	Hours
1	8
2	8
3	5
4	10
5	8
6	0
7	0
8	9
9	8
10	8
11	8
12	8
13	0
14	0
14 Days	80 Hours

Overtime owed: 3 hours (2 from day 4; 1 from day 8)

counted; rather, when the totals of daily overtime and over 80 differ, it is the higher that must apply.

The FLSA also specifies that only hours actually worked need to be counted toward determining overtime. That is, the organization is not required to include nonworked time such as vacation days, sick leave, holidays, and personal time as part of the 80 hours.

The "Regular Rate"

The so-named "regular rate" referred to in the FLSA includes the person's scheduled hourly rate plus on-call pay, call-in pay, and shift differential. Exhibit 1-3 presents an example of the effects of these additions on the rate.

Generally, hours spent at home on call are not counted as hours worked. This is generally the case because this treatment depends on the employee's freedom of movement while on call; often an argument can be made in favor of including on-call pay. In determining whether on-call time must be counted as hours worked, the government will generally look to determine whether the employee must remain on

Exhibit 1-2

"8 and 80" Example 2

Day	Hours
1	8
2	8
3	8
4	8
5	8
6	0
7	0
8	8
9	8
10	8
11	8
12	10
13	0
14	0
14 Days	82 Hours

Overtime owed: 2 hours (from day 12)

the employer's premises or be sufficiently close that the time cannot be used as the individual chooses. However, whether the hours on call are considered work time or not, *pay* received for such time is counted in determining the regular rate. Note also that when an employee who is on call is actually called in to perform work, the hours actually worked are counted in the total hours worked. If this is the case, the hours will be treated as working time for purposes of both minimum wage and overtime requirements.

Revised Overtime Eligibility Rules

In August 2004, the Bush administration introduced significant changes to the portions of the FLSA that address overtime, with the stated intent of helping an estimated 1.3 million low-wage workers while removing premium pay eligibility from certain higher paid employees.

Eligibility for overtime pay is one of the most frequently litigated workplace issues. The portions of the FLSA that address overtime pay and exemptions for professional,

Exhibit 1-3

"Regular Rate" Example

Overtime period: 7 days, 40 hours

Employee worked 50 hours, including 4 hours of call-in time

Rates paid: Basic: $14.00 per hour

              Shift differential: $1.00 per hour

              Call in: $65.00 (4 hours)

              On call: $40.00 (flat)

Calculation:		
$14.00 × 46 hours	=	$644.00
$1.00 × 46 hours	=	46.00
Call in	=	65.00
On call	=	40.00
Earning without overtime premium =		$795.00

$795.00/50 hours = $15.90 "regular rate"

One-half "regular rate" = $7.95

Premium: $7.95 × 10 hours	=	79.50
Total earned:	=	$802.95

administrative, and managerial employees affect tens of millions of workers, many of whom are paid hourly and are eligible for overtime pay. Some 25–30 million such workers held "managerial" or "administrative" jobs that fell into a broad gray area of the law and many of whom worked in excess of 40 hours per week at salaries that were low by contemporary standards. A long-standing attitude in business suggested a widespread belief that the person who worked in any supposed white-collar job need not be paid overtime.

The August 2004 changes, subsequently modified, specified that:

- Anyone earning less than $455 per week ($23,660 annually) is automatically qualified for overtime.
- Those earning more than $100,000 annually are not eligible for overtime *if* they "customarily and regularly perform at least one of the duties of an exempt executive, administrative, or professional employee identified in the standard tests of exemption." (As a result, there can be workers earning in excess of $100,000 who are eligible for overtime pay as long as they do not meet the foregoing qualification.)
- Certain workers, including police, firefighters and other first responders, practical nurses, health therapists, and certain veterans do not lose their eligibility.

How Well Do You Know the Wage and Hour Laws?

Some Managers' Questions

A sampling of questions asked concerning wage payment reveals that the majority of department managers have more concerns about overtime payment than any other wage and hour practices. The following questions and responses reflect many department managers' concerns about overtime.

Q—I have several hourly employees who frequently get busy around the middle of the shift and work right through their scheduled lunch break. How should this time be recorded? Can it cause overtime pay?

The time has to be recorded as time worked, and it has to drive overtime pay assuming it causes a person's total hours for the workweek to exceed 40. There is, however, a contradiction inherent in this practice: In most instances, permitting an employee to work an entire shift without a meal break is itself a violation of wage and hour law.

Q—I have an hourly employee who I discovered has regularly been taking work home to complete it. Are we supposed to pay for the time spent doing so? Can this practice cause overtime pay?

To answer both questions: Yes. The solution, of course, is to prohibit the taking home of work by nonexempt employees. However, one common problem associated with this practice is presented by the employee who takes work home without your knowledge and later claims pay for its completion. Your response should be, first, to let employees know they are not to take work home (nonexempt employees, that is—exempt employees can take home all the work they wish to), and second, to discipline those who act contrary to your instructions.

Many employees will take unfinished tasks home simply for the sake of getting them done or keeping up with the workload and will never make an issue of doing so. The danger resides with the occasional employee who may do so secretively for a period of time and then claim payment. This suggests that the manager must always be aware of each employee's level of output. Under wage and hour law, work done at home remains extra work for compensation purposes even if the manager is unaware it is being done.

Q—Should it not be enough for all employees to know that the organization has published rules for addressing overtime: rules that all can read and understand and comply with?

The rules are usually in the personnel policy manual and in the organization's employee handbook, and it is common for one of the most publicized overtime rules to require that all overtime must be approved in advance. However, a published rule does not get the organization off the hook for voluntary or casual overtime that has not received advance approval. The department manager must monitor such practices.

Q—A particular nonexempt employee regularly continues to work for 15–20 minutes after quitting time. Another puts in an extra 30 minutes every week or so without permission. Do we have to pay overtime in these circumstances?

Overtime payment is required under the law even if the employee does so without permission and in spite of a policy calling for advance approval. The organization is obligated to pay for all hours worked whether or not they occur in brief increments like 15 or 20 minutes and whether or not they are approved in advance. However, the department manager can discipline employees who put in extra time contrary to a policy calling for advance approval. The manager must also be aware of an obligation accruing for so-called casual overtime by an employee's habit of consistently clocking in early or clocking out late. The organization will likely have a policy requiring hourly employees to clock in or out within a certain amount of time (commonly anywhere from 6–15 minutes) before official starting time or after scheduled quitting time.

Q—I would like to schedule an occasional meeting over the lunch period, and have the staff bring their lunches. A colleague favors a once-per-week breakfast meeting held 1 hour before starting time. Do we have to pay extra for these practices?

Yes. For nonexempt employees, this is considered work time even though they may be consuming a meal while they listen or participate. As long as work is involved, it is work time. As long as the meeting is mandatory and business is discussed, for nonexempt employees, it is paid time.

Q—In my department, it is most convenient to have some employees take lunch at their workstations for the sake of telephone coverage and such. Is this acceptable?

This practice can be troublesome on two counts. First, the time must be counted as work time and it can drive overtime. Second, wage and hour law specifies that most employees' meal periods must consist of at least 30 minutes *uninterrupted by work*. Consider it a rule that when an employee is eating and working in the same time period, the time is always considered work time.

Q—How about the use of compensatory time for hourly employees instead of overtime?

This is generally not permitted. However, it is allowable under certain specific circumstances if the time off occurs within the same workweek as the extra time worked, and if the time off is granted at 1.5 times the extra worked time (e.g., 4 extra worked hours are compensated by 6 hours off). But this sort of "time-off plan" must be formalized in a written policy and the affected employees must agree to it.

Q—Can the employer reduce an exempt employee's pay for partial days missed?

No. Salaried—that is, exempt—employees are paid by the week or some other lengthier period, not by the hour. They are essentially paid for doing the job, not for working specific amounts of time. If they are docked for partial days, they could then be considered nonexempt and subject to the overtime provisions of the FLSA. The employer cannot have it both ways; that is, not paying for overtime but docking for hours missed. The DOL would rule that employees treated in this manner are nonexempt. An exempt employee who misses a *full* day of work can be docked for the day if all other applicable benefits (such as sick time, vacation, personal time, etc.) have been consumed.

Q—Is it generally acceptable for exempt employees to keep track of extra hours worked and thus accrue personal time or comp time to use later?

This is not acceptable under wage and hour law. Whether the exempt employee works 1 hour or 16 hours on any particular day, the pay for the day remains the same.

Q—For the sake of building a team and helping establish solid interpersonal relationships, I would like to hold an occasional breakfast or dinner gathering. Attendance would be voluntary and no business would be conducted. The sole purpose would be to get to know each other better. Is this allowable, or would we have to pay people for their time?

If attendance is truly voluntary and no business is conducted, you will have no obligation to pay for their time.

The Manager's Timekeeping Responsibilities

What the department manager will be required to do for timekeeping purposes may vary according to the particular organization's payroll system and the numbers of exempt and nonexempt employees in the department. In general, in monitoring employees' time and properly addressing payroll system requirements, the first-line manager will be expected to:

- Carefully review each time record for calculation errors or other discrepancies between hours worked and what has been recorded. (This record may involve a time sheet completed manually, a time card punched at a clock, or an electronic entry into an automated attendance system.)

- Properly note break times and meal periods as required by the payroll system and ensure that all time recorded is in the appropriate place (for the correct day or shift).

- Ensure that worked overtime has been properly approved, and address any employee time-recording practices that could result in so-called casual overtime.

- Ensure that employees do not place extraneous entries or notations on the time record. Time records should be for recording time worked only and should not be used for relaying messages or explaining entries.

- Periodically remind employees of appropriate time-recording practices. It would be helpful to make this a topic at an occasional department meeting.

- Let any affected employee know up-front (that is, before paychecks are issued) that he or she might not be paid for certain absences or under certain exceptional circumstances.

- Ensure that all time records for the department are completed, checked for accuracy, and submitted by the deadline called for by the payroll system.

Conscientious Control of Overtime Required

Monitoring Is Essential

In many departments, overtime is similar to absenteeism in one critical dimension: It tends to go out of control or at least increase if it seems as though no one is watching or no one cares. Although overtime is usually a component of the department's budget, it can nevertheless get out of control if not closely monitored.

Overtime Is Not Always the Answer

For some occasional needs, overtime, even recognizing payment at time-and-a-half, is more economical and more practical than adding staff. But if a particular need continues indefinitely, it is often worth considering the addition of staff or the addition of hours for certain part-time employees. Overtime should be considered a short-term solution; it should rarely be used to fill a well-known recurring need that can be more economically addressed with other staffing options. The situation to be avoided is one in which an employee receives steady overtime to a point at which the overtime payment becomes regarded as part of the person's regular income.

Causes of Overtime

The causes of overtime can be many and varied, but within the organization that is experiencing excessive overtime use, the causes often include most or all of the following:

- *Variations in workload*. The variations in workload most often prompting overtime are those due to unexpected changes in demand, unanticipated alterations of deadlines, and genuine emergency situations. Since variations of this nature are not predictable, overtime is often the only recourse.
- *Absenteeism*. There is often a demonstrable, direct relationship between employee absenteeism and the need for overtime. Absenteeism increases and the requests for overtime increase, especially in patient-care and other direct-service activities where the one-for-one replacement of absent staff is essential.
- *Toleration of substandard performance*. An attitude of passivity sometimes permeates management and workforce alike. All parties come to accept that work not accomplished on regular time will be done on overtime, and thus by default, a practice develops of rewarding substandard performance.
- *General acceptance of overtime as a normal practice rather than an exception*. If the prevailing attitude has always been that overtime is available to catch up, then overtime will always be depended upon to do so. There often appears to be some validity to the notion that work expands to consume the time available for its completion.

- *Lack of management accountability.* If the first-line manager does not have to answer to an immediate superior for the use of overtime without particular concern for its cost, overtime will come to be accepted as normal and thus will be less likely to be seen as a way of addressing handling true exceptions.
- *Rigid scheduling practices.* When the manager or scheduler is constrained so severely by scheduling practices so as to be unable to schedule without causing overtime in cyclic schedules, an implied guarantee of overtime has been extended to elements of the workforce. Built-in overtime, and indeed all forms of guaranteed overtime, undermine the basic purposes of overtime and again lead toward its acceptance as a normal practice.
- *Bargaining unit work rules.* Various labor contracts state that only certain classifications of employees can perform certain kinds of work. Often under such rules, the logical persons to meet unforeseen requirements, such as part-time employees who could have their hours temporarily increased, are prevented from being used most efficiently because the contract may state, for example, that overtime must be offered first to full-time employees by order of seniority.
- *Inappropriate or insufficient equipment and inefficient physical work area.* Physical conditions that increase worker fatigue or impede the efficient performance of work often make it necessary to catch up using overtime. When it comes to productivity, an employee can be only as efficient as the equipment and the work environment will allow.

Toward Effective Control of Overtime

There are several approaches available to the first-line manager for controlling overtime while minimizing the risk of running afoul of the FLSA. These include the following.

Regulating Demand

In some departments (there are a number of functions within a healthcare organization to which this cannot apply), it is possible to take actions that regulate the demand for the department's services. Means available for the regulating demand include working on a reservation or appointment basis, promoting low-demand periods, and using complementary scheduling when it may be possible to schedule certain kinds of users into certain time periods.

Improving Staffing Practices

Among the steps the manager can consider to improve the department's staffing practices and thus help reduce overtime are cross-training employees of equivalent skill and grade in each other's jobs; using float personnel as appropriate; utilizing per diem, casual, or optional staff; increasing the hours of certain part-time employees; and constantly reevaluating scheduling practices to assure that they recognize the reality of the department's staffing circumstances.

Analyze and Improve Work Methods

Ineffective work methods; inadequate operating procedures; ineffective, obsolete, or otherwise inappropriate equipment; and inefficient workplace layout all tend to depress productivity and thus increase the pressure for overtime. Look closely at the backlog of work and bottleneck situations that seem to necessitate periodic overtime.

Control Absenteeism

As suggested earlier, there is often a direct relationship between a department's level of absenteeism and the amount of overtime worked. To address absenteeism directly is to directly address the problem of excess overtime as well.

Manage Responsibly

Managing responsibly includes accepting accountability for the amount of overtime usage in the department. Such acceptance suggests a thorough, rational approach to the examination of each instance of possible overtime. When possible overtime need arises, before granting approval, check first to determine whether the work can be postponed, reassigned to persons who are already present, or accomplished by faster, more efficient means. If these solutions are unavailable, check for available part-time, float, or call-in help. Consider also available full-time staff who have been absent part of the week. Under the strict FLSA requirement to pay overtime for hours in excess of 40 (and in the absence of the occasionally encountered organizational policy for overtime payment for more than 8 hours in a day), employees who have been absent for part of a week are often willing to make up all or part of the balance of the workweek by working at their regular rates.

Only upon exhausting all of the foregoing possibilities without resolution should the manager authorize overtime, and only then according to organizational policies that are consistent with the overtime portions of the FLSA.

Overtime Authorization

First-line managers often experience problems with the authorization of overtime. Many organizations' systems call for approval in advance. However, because of emergency situations, advance authorization is not always possible, and employees who may be put in a position of having to judge for themselves should know the applicable rules.

To cite an illustration, a process reflected in one particular organization's overtime pay guidelines includes the following concerning authorization:

1. Scheduled (anticipated) overtime shall be approved in advance by the department manager.

2. Unscheduled overtime shall be handled as follows:
   - An employee who determines that it may be necessary to work beyond the assigned shift must make a good-faith effort to obtain the department manager's approval.
   - Unscheduled overtime worked without advance authorization shall be reviewed for approval on a daily basis. The department manager shall initial the time record to indicate approval.
   - Overtime payment shall not be permitted to result from employees' card-punching practices. Employees not engaged in overtime work shall punch in and out according to timekeeping practices.

Constant Visibility

A significant part of the control of overtime consists of maintaining overtime in a position of prominence and paying attention to its importance. One way of keeping overtime visible in the department is to publicize, on a regular basis, the department's performance against budget in its use of overtime. If overtime is not a separately budgeted item (although in most organizations it is), then at budget preparation time, the manager should strongly suggest that overtime be made a budget subaccount in its own right and that actual overtime be reported back against budgeted overtime on the regular budget-reporting cycle.

Another method for keeping the overtime issue visible involves the use of an organization-wide overtime committee. The experience of one organization proved interesting, and since the approach was not particularly unique, similar results have likely been experienced elsewhere: An overtime committee was formed during a year in which overtime appears to have gone completely out of control. Consisting of a dozen or more people—administration, finance, human resources, and the heads of various departments—the committee wrestled with the causes of overtime and the overtime approval process, and watched overtime usage diminish until it was within budget limits. When the problem went away and the committee began to meet less often and eventually not at all, overtime again increased. However, each time the committee was reconstituted in response to rising overtime, overtime immediately began to track downward. Thus, visible attention paid to overtime is often sufficient to impress people with its importance so they become more careful.

If a department is properly staffed, it will likely experience some legitimate overtime needs from time to time. Overtime will always be subject to a certain amount of abuse or at least questionable use, and abuse and misuse are likely to increase if it is not made plain that overtime is subject to constant monitoring. Even if the problem is resolved periodically, it is likely to recur. The only long-run solution to the control of overtime is an appropriate level of constant attention and active monitoring and control by first-line management.

A Manager's Advantage

Although the largest part of wage and hour legislation is of greater concern to others in the organization, such as human resources and finance (specifically the payroll section), it is nevertheless to the department manager's advantage to understand how and why employees are classified as they are and how elements of their compensation, particularly overtime, are determined. Human resources and the payroll department may be the experts concerning some aspects of wage and hour law, but they cannot top the perspective of the department manager. The first-line manager is among the staff, on the floor where the work is done and where most of the action takes place. A knowledgeable department manager can help keep the organization out of trouble concerning employee classifications (exempt versus nonexempt), help minimize pay discrepancies with conscientious timekeeping, and help keep the budget in line through the active control of overtime.

Questions for Review and Discussion

1. Why are the employees working in some positions that clearly qualify as exempt positions nevertheless paid overtime?

2. Do you believe it is allowable to maintain two different definitions of the workweek in the same organization? Why or why not?

3. Why should the organization have an enforceable policy limiting the amount of time during which an employee must clock in and limiting the time during which the employee must clock out after the shift?

4. Identify the principal reasons prompting the initial passage of the Fair Labor Standards Act.

5. What are the essential differences between the executive and administrative exempt-employee classifications?

6. What are some of the ways in which employee classification information may be constructively applied?

7. What conditions would have to be met for an hourly employee titled secretary to be legitimately made exempt with the title of administrative assistant?

8. Under what conditions can you hold a before or after work gathering of your employees without being liable for overtime payment?

9. Is it lawful to allow your employee group to shorten their workday by working through a meal period if they all agree to the practice in writing? Why or why not?

10. Describe at least two sets of circumstances under which an employee's on-call hours must be counted as worked hours.

Chapter 2

The Health Insurance Portability and Accountability Act (HIPAA): Not All About Health Insurance

Joan M. Kiel, PhD, CHPS, *Chairman University HIPAA Compliance and Associate Professor HMS, Duquesne University, Pittsburgh, Pennsylvania*

Chapter Objectives

- Develop an understanding of the circumstances leading to the passage of Health Insurance Portability and Accountability Act (HIPAA) and the several purposes that HIPAA is intended to serve.
- Examine the portions of HIPAA that are most pertinent to working managers, specifically the significant sections of the second of the five titles of HIPAA referred to in legislation as Administrative Simplification.
- Facilitate familiarization with the rules applicable in the implementation of HIPAA.
- Define the manager's role relative to the HIPAA Privacy Rule and Security Rules.
- Review the responsibilities incumbent upon the organization for the implementation of HIPAA and its maintenance as standard operating procedure.
- Review the potential uses of personal patient health information by the organization and define the circumstances governing the release of such information.

Introduction

The Health Insurance Portability and Accountability Act (HIPAA) is an important piece of federal legislation that has changed the way healthcare organizations do business. When it was initially being debated, healthcare managers feared the worst, thinking of added expenses. They surmised that they would have to add staff, and they thought that patients would be upset. Through it all, healthcare managers have had to make adjustments in operations and keep abreast of HIPAA. This chapter details HIPAA and describes how a healthcare manager can successfully implement the pertinent portions of this law.

History and Rationale

What patients tell physicians can sometimes consist of some of the most confidential information that pertains to themselves. They tell it to physicians with the understanding that it will be used for their medical care and will not be passed on to others who are not involved in their care. Unfortunately, this essential confidentiality is not always observed. Consider the following examples: Information discussed by a physician and a physical therapist in a less-than-private setting is overheard by visitors leaving the adjacent office of a social worker; written information is left on a computer screen in an open nursing station when a nurse answers a call light; or information is used for financial gain when facts about a well-known patient is sold to a tabloid publication. Additionally, information stored electronically has the potential to be sent to many people with the click of a computer stroke, necessitating the implementation of security systems to prevent "healthcare hacking." Whether perpetrated purposefully or inadvertently, scenarios such as those discussed has led to federal legislation to protect patient health information.

HIPAA was enacted in part to protect the privacy, security, and confidentiality of patient health information. It also ensures secure transactions and assigns identifiers for providers, insurers, and patients to ease administrative transactions. HIPAA exists for both for the patient and the healthcare delivery system so that confidential information is utilized as it should be for the care of the patient and so that administrative transactions can be completed effectively and efficiently.

HIPAA, or Public Law 104-191, contains five titles addressing various areas of responsibility:

1. Healthcare Access, Portability, and Renewability
2. A. Preventing Healthcare Fraud and Abuse
   B. Medical Liability Reform
   C. Administrative Simplification
3. Tax-Related Health Provision
4. Group Health Plan Requirements
5. Revenue Offsets

Contained within the Administrative Simplification section of Title II are the three main areas that are pertinent to most healthcare managers: electronic data interchange, which includes transactions, identifiers, and code sets; privacy; and security. To further delineate these three main areas, HIPAA is divided into 11 rules. It is from these rules that healthcare managers then develop policies and procedures to ensure compliance with the law.

The 11 Rules of HIPAA

The first portion of HIPAA, Transactions and Code Sets, was scheduled for compliance by October 16, 2002. As of October 16, 2009, just 6 of the 11 rules of HIPAA had been released for implementation with compliance dates. Thus, for healthcare managers, HIPAA implementation will be an ongoing process for some time to come. The 11 rules are as follows:

1. The **Claims Attachment Standards Rule** establishes national standards for the format and content of electronic claims attachment transactions (proposed in the September 23, 2005 Federal Register).
2. The **Clinical Data Rules/Electronic Signature Standard** establishes national standards for clinical data and data transmission.
3. The **Data Security Rule** establishes physical, technical, and administrative protocols for the security and integrity of electronic health data (April 20, 2005).
4. The **Enforcement Rule** establishes rules for how the government intends to enforce HIPAA (February 15, 2006).
5. The **Standard Transaction for First Report of Injury Rule** establishes national standards for the format and content of electronic first-report-of-injury transactions used in Workers' Compensation cases.
6. The **Standard Unique Identifier for Employers Rule** establishes the federal tax identification number as an employer's national unique identifier (July 30, 2004).
7. The **Unique Identifier for Individuals Rule** mandates a single patient identifier for all of an individual's patient health information.
8. The **Standard Unique National Health Plan/Payer Identifier Rule** establishes a national identifier for each health insurer.
9. The **Standard Unique Healthcare Provider Identifier Rule** establishes a national identifier for each provider (May 23, 2007).
10. The **Privacy Rule** establishes guidelines for the use and disclosure of patient health information (April 14, 2003).
11. The **Transactions and Code Sets Rule** establishes standard formats and coding of electronic claims and related transactions (October 16, 2002 or 2003).[1]

A Manager's Guide to the HIPAA Rules

As healthcare managers had just passed beyond the Y2K flurry of activity, the first rule of HIPAA, Transactions and Code Sets, was being released for implementation. The required implementation date was October 16, 2002, although covered entities were able to request a 1-year extension. As part of HIPAA's mission to ease electronic transactions, this rule focused on the development of standardized formats for electronic claims and their related transactions. HIPAA also specified what a HIPAA transaction was.

1. Healthcare claims or equivalent transactions
2. Healthcare payment and remittance advice
3. Coordination of benefits
4. Healthcare claim status
5. Enrollment and disenrollment in a health plan
6. Eligibility for a health plan
7. Health plan premium payments
8. Referral certification and authorization
9. First report of injury
10. Health claims attachments
11. Other transactions that the secretary may prescribe by regulation[2]

Healthcare managers need to be aware that as the revised *International Classification of Diseases (ICD-10)* is introduced (projected for Fall 2011), these transactions may undergo some changes. But all have the common objective of facilitating more accurate and efficient transactions.

The next rule to be implemented came with much fanfare (as opposed to the Transactions and Code Sets, which arrived quietly), as it impacted patients directly. With Transactions and Code Sets, patients do not know how their medical diagnoses are being coded, nor is it a great concern to them (as long as the bill is paid by the insurer). With the Privacy Rule, however, patients have forms to sign and new policies to adhere to with regard to accessing their health information.

The covered entity must employ an individual designated as a privacy officer. This person can be full time or part time, but must be intimately knowledgeable of HIPAA. It is certainly not a position to be given to someone in title only. This person is responsible for understanding and implementing the Privacy Rule. Although no specific background is required of the privacy officer, the person must have an understanding of health information, information technology, regulatory compliance, and management.

The first big change for both the staff and the patients was the introduction of the Notice of Health Information Privacy Practice, simply called the Notice. Employees of the covered entity have been required to provide the Notice once to every patient seen on or after April 14, 2003. On February 17, 2009, the Health Information

Technology for Economic and Clinical Health Act (HITECH) made changes to the Notice; thus on and after February 17, 2010, the revised Notice must be provided to all patients once. This is to be remembered concerning the HIPAA Privacy Rule: Whenever the Notice is revised by any legislation, it must again be provided to all patients.[3] It is necessary to have a process in place, whether paper or electronic, to keep track of who has been given the Notice and who has not. For example, if a long-standing patient does not present at the office again until 2012, the system must indicate that this patient has not been in since before February 17, 2010 and thus must receive the revised Notice. On the other hand, one should not wish to waste time and money or irritate the patients by repeatedly giving them the Notice. The Notice must also be changed on the provider's website and in any postings within the facility. Managers must also budget for the costs of keeping the Notice current.

Patients will also see new forms when they request copies of their medical information. The Privacy Rule has altered the standard Release of Information Form, although it remains unchanged in its essential contents. Patients also have the opportunity to request to amend their medical records, and forms must be completed for this purpose. Once completed, forms are reviewed by the author of the medical record notes or perhaps others if the original writer is not available. The privacy officer must be able to lead this process and ensure that all HIPAA documents are retained for 6 years. This in itself takes planning as one must decide whether records will be stored on-site or off-site, and electronically or on paper. A sample request form is shown in Exhibit 2-1.

Not all information is to be retained. Material that is not to be kept must be disposed of in a manner that ensures it cannot reasonably be reproduced. For paper, the most popular disposal method is shredding. For electronic data, the most popular way is degaussing. For either method, however, the covered entity must have a policy in place. If an external firm is used for disposal, it must provide the covered entity with certificates of destruction stating that they did in fact destroy the data and did not retain it or pass it on to others. A certificate of external destruction is shown in Exhibit 2-2.

A significant requirement that encompasses the entire covered entity involves the knowledge and awareness of HIPAA by all workforce members. All must be trained about HIPAA, and that training must be documented. In addition to training, HIPAA awareness must be routinely reinforced. This provision was put in place so that HIPAA is not forgotten, but rather remains a part of standard operating procedures. At every staff meeting the healthcare manager can simply have HIPAA on the agenda and review its status and implementation. The manager can review with the privacy officer how processes and procedures are being carried out and what their apparent effects are on the entity.

Employees must also be aware of their limits on access to information. Based on one's role, employees will be allowed to have access to only the information they need to fulfill their roles and nothing more. The need to know and minimum necessary standards apply such that employees do not acquire patient health information over and above what is needed to complete the task at hand.

Exhibit 2-1

Request for Amendment of Health Information

Patient name: _____

Medical record number: _____

Birth date: _____

Address: _____

Date of information to be amended: _____

Type of information to be amended: _____

Why is the information inaccurate or incomplete? _____

_____

_____

What should the information say? _____

_____

_____

If the request is agreed upon, where else should the amended information go?

Name: _____

Address: _____

_____   _____
Signature of patient   Date

To Be Completed by the Healthcare Provider:

Date received: _____

By whom: _____

Request for amendment has been: ACCEPTED   DENIED

If denied, state reason: _____

_____

Information is accurate and complete

Healthcare provider's reason: _____

_____

_____

_____

_____

_____   _____
Signature of healthcare provider   Date

Exhibit 2-2

Destruction of Patient Health Information by an External Entity

Name of facility and address: _____

Vendor name and address: _____

Description of information, and time period of the information: _____

Pick-up date of material: _____

Quantity of information destroyed: _____

Date of destruction: _____

Method of destruction: _____

Name of person doing destruction: _____

Signature: _____ Date: _____

As stated in the Notice of Health Information Privacy Practices, a patient has the right to file a HIPAA compliant with the covered entity, usually directly with the privacy officer. The first duty of the privacy officer—and this is where that official really needs to know HIPAA thoroughly—is to determine whether the complaint is truly HIPAA related. The patient cannot use the HIPAA complaint process, for example, to complain about waiting too long to see a physician. The covered entity must have a complaint process in place directing where and how patients can file complaints to how these are to be investigated and processed. If a complaint is warranted, sanctions must be assessed against the involved employees.

Not only do complaints warrant follow-up, but routine HIPAA audits may also reveal something that is not HIPAA compliant. Although the HIPAA Privacy Rule does not specify how often audits are to be performed, the healthcare manager can base HIPAA audit frequency on the timing of other audits such as those for billing and quality assurance. Areas in which issues arise are of course audited more frequently. It is necessary to document the audits and their findings; any adverse findings must be addressed via a documented action plan with subsequent follow-up on results.

Healthcare managers need to work with their privacy officer in relation to two external groups: business associates and researchers. Business associates are external constituents who see the covered entities personal health information but are not part of the organization's workforce (e.g., a computer vendor or an outside billing company). With such associates there must be a signed business-associate agreement calling for compliance with all HIPAA regulations. Under HITECH, implemented February 17, 2010, business associates must adhere to all of the HIPAA Security policies and not simply provide reasonable assurance that they are keeping patient health information private, secure, and confidential. The covered entity must also remain in communication with business associates to ensure that any noncompliance is corrected immediately and is not as a result of malice.

Persons conducting research in your organization and using personal health information also must be compliant with HIPAA. Data used for research cannot compromise the privacy, security, and confidentiality of patient health information.

The healthcare manager, in concert with the HIPAA privacy officer, must be proactive in protecting patient health information. Whether involving house staff, patients, themselves, business associates, or researchers, there is always much to be attended to and monitored under the HIPAA Privacy Rule.

Following the Privacy Rule is the HIPAA Security Rule, implemented April 20, 2005. The Security Rule is unique in including both required and addressable policies, thus it is entity dependent. Covered entities must follow the implementation specifications for the required policies. With the addressable policies, a covered entity must assess whether each implementation specification is reasonable and appropriate for protecting its patient health information.[3] The policies are then further divided into the three categories of technical, administrative, and physical aspects of security.

Just as the Privacy Rule calls for a privacy officer, a security officer is required for the Security Rule. This can be the same person as the privacy officer, as long as the individual has the time and expertise to cover both roles. Employees must be trained in security measures and this training must be documented. Security awareness among employees must also be stressed throughout the organization.

Documentation is vital concerning the Security Rule. Just as with privacy documentation, all HIPAA security documentation must be retained for 6 years. The Security Rule also necessitates a disaster manual documenting procedures to follow in the event of a disaster during which health information could be in jeopardy. This manual should exist in concert with the emergency-mode-operation plan intended to keep the organization functioning to the best of its ability in any compromised situation. The security officer, often the primary author of the manual, must be thoroughly conversant with its contents at all times. The security officer will most likely also be the person who implements the security incident policy. Table 2-1 lists the necessary security policies.

Table 2-1 *Areas of Necessary Security Policy Coverage*

Security Policies	Administrative	Physical	Technical
Required	1. Risk Analysis/Assessment 2. Risk Management 3. Sanction Policy/Disciplinary System 4. IS Activity Review 5. Assigned Security Responsibility (Security Officer) 6. Workforce/Personnel Security 7. Clearinghouse Functions/ Hybrid Entity 8. Response and Reporting 9. Data Backup Plan 10. Security Plan 11. Critical Business Processes/ Contingency Plan 12. Business Associates 13. Evaluation	1. Workstation Security 2. Device and Media Controls 3. Disposal of Computers 4. Media Reuse	1. Unique User Identification 2. Emergency Access 3. Audit Trails 4. Person or Entity Authentication
Addressable	1. Authorization and/or Supervision of Access to personal health information Personal Health Information (PHI) 2. Access to Data/Workforce Clearance 3. Terminating Access 4. Granting Access/Access Control 5. Access Establishment and Modification/Personnel Security 6. Security Reminders/Awareness 7. Malicious Software 8. Log-in Monitoring 9. Password Management 10. Testing and Revision 11. Applications and Data Criticality	1. Disaster Recovery/ Restore Lost Data 2. Physical Safeguards 3. Access Control & Validation 4. Maintenance Records/Logs 5. Accountability/ Transfer of Media & 6. Copy electronic personal health information.	1. Automatic Log Off 2. Encryption and Decryption Mechanism 3. Authentication of Electronic PHI 4. Integrity Controls 5. Encryption of Transmitted PHI

The security officer must be the person who implements and monitors policy compliance. The HIPAA Rule does not prescribe specific security measures, but rather provides blanket mandates and allows the organization to decide how these will be met. For example, the organization must have authentication methods in place, but whether these include passwords, thumbprints, or retinal scans is the organization's decision.[3]

Since access to patient health information is role-based, access-control audits must be completed. Employees who do not need access to information to perform their jobs will be identified on an audit if they violate access rights. With electronic records violations are readily detectable as one can look at the computer history, but with paper records there is more reliance on one's word that another was seen with the record. Computers should clearly record that electronic records are audited when one logs in. The computer should also have an automatic log-off process in the event of an emergency. Employees should never share their passwords except in a true emergency, nor should they store their passwords in obvious places.

When an employee leaves the organization either voluntarily or involuntarily, access must be terminated. It is particularly important when an employee is terminated involuntarily, as time is of the essence to prevent the terminated employee from saving any files for personal use or destroying files. If at all possible, a terminated employee's computer should be examined for any such activity before the person's departure. Thus another function of the security officer or designee is to have all files backed up as a precaution against loss.

In the same manner as the privacy officer, the security officer needs to manage the business-associate agreements. The same method used with the Privacy Rule can be used here.

Although the Security Rule is fairly extensive, its presence it is not nearly as evident to the patient as is the Privacy Rule.

The final three rules, the Standard Unique Employer Identifier Rule, the National Provider Identifier Rule, and the Enforcement Rule are not as extensive as the Privacy and Security Rules but they are just as important from a managerial perspective. The Standard Unique Employer Identifier Rule was implemented July 30, 2004. This rule calls for the organization to use its employer identification number (EIN) as its standard identifier. Many organizations were already doing this before HIPAA, so compliance was not an issue. For those who were not doing so, it was a matter of replacing what they had been previously using with the EIN.

The National Provider Identifier Rule was implemented May 23, 2007. This rule required healthcare providers to use a 10-digit unique identifier. The covered entities had to apply for the numbers and ensure they were used in all transactions. Computer fields, as well as forms, and policies needed to be updated. Inventorying the locations where the numbers are used is itself a large task.

The Enforcement Rule was implemented on February 16, 2006. As its name indicates, this rule mandates enforcement of HIPAA. Healthcare managers had to develop appropriate policies and procedures. This rule specifies what happens if there is a violation of HIPAA; it describes the issues of evidence and trial situations. Mangers need to understand this rule in the unlikely event of ever being a defendant or a plaintiff or involved in some other way in a legal debate.

These six rules of HIPAA currently set the stage for the remaining five rules. The healthcare manager will utilize the same skills and processes in implementing the remaining five as applied in the implementation of the first six. Most importantly, managers must come to view HIPAA as a part of standard operating procedures.

What Organizations Need to Do for All Six Implemented Parts

With 6 of the 11 rules of HIPAA released and 5 more to go, healthcare managers need to see HIPAA as an essential part of general operations. If its inevitability is recognized and it is incorporated into how one regularly does business, it will not feel like a legal albatross. Its integration into standard operating procedure requires putting some specific things in place.

First, as stated for the Privacy and Security Rules, a covered entity must employ a privacy officer and a security officer. Once in place, this person or persons can then, in concert with the healthcare manager, implement and manage HIPAA. A sample job description for a privacy officer appears in Exhibit 2-3.

The privacy and security officer is supported by a HIPAA committee. The HIPAA committee is comprised of people from information technology, health information management, administration, human resources, finance, and research if applicable. All of the parts of HIPAA must be represented on the HIPAA committee and thus a wide variety is needed in the committee's membership.

The third and most time-consuming responsibility is the development of the policies and procedures needed for all of the HIPAA rules. These policies are best developed from the law itself rather than from secondary sources. In this manner, the organization will be using the most precise policy language. Also, as with the Security Rule's address-able policies, all organizations will not be the same in size and scope so it is preferable to avoid using policies from other organizations. Each HIPAA rule should be covered by a policy manual or at least a separate manual section for easy reference. In drafting one's own, the organization will also be able to include consideration of implementation and changes to business operations. The HIPAA committee can be most helpful in drafting polices. In addition, many organizations have a policy committee that can also assist.

The fourth responsibility requires the covered entity to provide a training and awareness program for all workforce members. Not only as each part of HIPAA is un-veiled must there be training, but this training must also be ingrained into the fabric of the organization. It cannot be a do-it-once and forget-about-it event. Training can be done in-house or outsourced; it can be done face-to-face, via computer, or by distance education. In the majority of small- to medium-sized organizations, it is the role of the privacy and security officers to perform this task. In larger organizations, online training is used or is outsourced to trainers so that it will not take up all of the time

Exhibit 2-3

Sample Job Description, Privacy Officer

Title: Privacy Officer
Division: Corporate Administration
Reports to: Chief Executive Officer of the covered entity
Position purpose: The privacy officer is responsible and accountable for all activities related to the development, implementation, evaluation, and modification of activities concerning the privacy of and access to patient health information as designated by HIPAA.

Position responsibilities:

- Identify, implement, and maintain organizational patient health information privacy policies and procedures.
- Work with the security officer, compliance committee, management, and staff in ensuring that privacy and security policies and procedures are maintained.
- Is responsible and accountable for all activities related to the privacy of and access to patient health information.
- Perform health information privacy risk assessments.
- Perform ongoing compliance monitoring activities and works with management to operationalize these monitoring activities into the daily functions.
- Develop and implement compliance related forms.
- Develop and maintain initial and ongoing training for all workforce members of the organization on HIPAA and HITECH.
- Review and bring into compliance all business associate agreements in regards to HIPAA and HITECH.
- Establish and implement a system to track assess to patient health information.
- Establish and implement a process allowing patients the right to inspect and request to amend their health information.
- Establish a program whereby complaints can be received, documented, tracked, and investigated.
- Develop a disciplinary system of sanctions for failure to comply with HIPAA for employees and constituents of the organization.
- Promote an ongoing culture of information privacy awareness and compliance to all related policies and laws.
- Develop policies and procedures for release of information and access to information.

- Maintain current knowledge of applicable federal, state, local, and organizational privacy laws and regulations.
- Work with all facilities and departments to standardize policies and procedures in regards to the privacy of patient health information.
- Lead the compliance committee and amend it as needed.
- Communicate as often as necessary due to changing regulations and compliance issues.
- Perform other activities as assigned.

Position qualifications:

- Bachelor's degree in a healthcare-related field is required.
- Certification in Healthcare Privacy and Security is recommended.
- Three years of management experience in health care.
- Knowledge of information privacy laws and issues related to access to health information, release of information, and patient rights.

of the privacy and security officers. All of the training must be documented and the documentation must be retained for 6 years. Some more thoughtful managers simply put it in the employee files and keep it beyond 6 years as long as the person remains employed. Training is done as changes occur to HIPAA, but sustained awareness must to be a regular business practice. Simply having a discussion at a staff meeting on HIPAA may constitute awareness; therefore, this activity need not be extensive to be effective. Of course if there is a violation, training must address that in the correction plan. Training is never ending, as HIPAA itself must be regarded as never ending.

The fifth responsibility concerns the development of a document retention system to retain all HIPAA materials for a minimum of 6 years. At the onset, many thought that this would be easy: Simply save everything. But doing so eventually becomes overwhelming in the face of the need to retrieve a specific record, thus the need for an organized method of retention.

HIPAA materials that must be retained include the forms that patients, employees, and business associates complete, policies that are revised, employee records such as for training and sanctions, audits and updates, and any material that contains patient health information that may not exist in the formal medical record (e.g., research forms). As a first step, a documentation retention subcommittee of the HIPAA committee can be formed. It is this group's responsibility to determine what needs to be retained and who has it, and then determine the quantity of information to save and whether its form be paper, electronic, or audio. Multiply that effort by 6 years and then determine how and where the material can be saved. For example, can paper be scanned? Or will the paper be saved in hard copy but perhaps off-site? Here budgetary considerations emerge. Initially many managers did not consider processing and retention costs; the amount of material that must be saved can be large. Also, if one contracts with an off-site storage organization, it is necessary to reckon with the cost of retrieval. How much per piece? How much per retrieval trip? Retention is not simply saving items; it necessarily includes an understanding of the process of doing business.

The sixth responsibility concerns development and implementation of an audit system. This was much more prominent when the Enforcement Rule was implemented. The basic assumption is that if it is not documented, it was not done. Unfortunately, one's word is never good enough when the healthcare manager must respond to a HIPAA complaint. Making audits a part of standard operating procedures shows that the organization is serious about it, and that, in itself, helps create a culture of caring and competency. A sample audit report form is shown in Exhibit 2-4.

Exhibit 2-4

Sample Audit Report Form

Date of audit: _____

Audit performed by: _____

Subject of audit: **Please circle subject of audit**
                    Computer log-ins
                    Medical record documentation
                    Coding and billing (claim denials)
                    Adherence to confidentiality policies
                    Adherence to security policies
                    Update of employee files
                    HIPAA training of employees
                    Review of violations/operational issues
                    Review of personnel access to patient health information
                    Number of breach of confidentiality issues
                    Claim denials
                    Other: _____

Department audit took place in: _____

Sample of employees surveyed: Number: _____   Type: _____

Adherence percentage: _____

Nonadherence percentage: _____

Report rationale: _____

Action plan:

_____

_____

The next responsibility calls for development and posting of a complaint process. Any patient has the right to file a HIPAA complaint if he or she believes that something that occurred is not consistent with HIPAA requirements. This must be clearly stated in the notice, which must also delineate the process for filing a complaint both internally and with the federal government. The healthcare manager must take every complaint seriously and ensure it is investigated. The manager, along with the HIPAA privacy officer, must first determine if a complaint is actually HIPAA related. If so, the privacy officer will further investigate and also call in the security officer if the complaint involves security issues. If not HIPAA related, the complaint goes back to the manager for follow-up as a general personnel issue. Complaints must be tracked such that employee follow-up occurs, it is determined that office procedures are altered to prevent further complaints as necessary, and training is reinforced in common complaint areas.

The final major responsibility, the sanction process, functions in concert with the complaint process. Although HIPAA does not specify the nature of the sanctions, the organization must apply reasonable sanctions that are consistent with the seriousness of the violations. It must be noted, however, that a violation of HIPAA can also provoke civil and criminal penalties; therefore, all violations and sanctions must be taken seriously. Sanctions can include termination of an offending employee and additional penalties. It is absolutely necessary that the manager retain documentation establishing that the employee was trained and did attend awareness meetings. It is unreasonable to expect the employees to observe HIPAA regulations if they have not been adequately trained. A sample of a form for documenting training appears as Exhibit 2-5.

In many organizations, HIPAA training documentation is kept with general employee training records and is maintained by the HR department. No matter who maintains the records, however, the HIPAA privacy and security officers remain accountable for training employees on the HIPAA Privacy and Security Rules.

Exhibit 2-5

HIPAA Training Record

Name: _____

Employee identification number: _____

Department: _____

Employment start date: _____

Date	Training Topic	Comments
____	_____	_____
____	_____	_____
____	_____	_____

Keeping Up with HIPAA

With six of the eleven rules of HIPAA implemented, healthcare managers have much to do. As seen with HITECH and its influence the HIPAA Privacy and Security Rules, while managers await the next five rules, they must also remain current with the original six. When HIPAA is essentially up and running in the organization, this task of keeping up to date becomes less daunting. Managers are encouraged to attend conferences, join professional associations, read the literature, and foster awareness of HIPAA throughout their organizations.

Questions for Review and Discussion

1. Under HIPAA are patients allowed to alter their health information records? If so, how must this be done?

2. Why is documentation of HIPAA training necessary?

3. Define the term "business associate" and describe how and by whom the activities of such associates are controlled.

4. What are the circumstances that primarily govern anyone's access to a patient's personal medical information?

5. What is the purpose of the Health Information Technology Economic and Clinical Health Act (HITECH) implemented February 17, 2010?

6. What do you believe have been the biggest objections to HIPAA voiced by managers and administrators?

7. So far, what seem to have been the greatest visible effects of HIPAA?

8. Describe the form or forms in which a covered organization must maintain its HIPAA records.

9. What do you consider to be the primary reasons for the enactment of HIPAA?

10. What is the general legal attitude toward the absence of documentation needed to resolve a complaint or respond to a challenge?

References

1. Mossman, V. S. (2006). Recap of HIPAA information sessions and guidelines. *Action Newsletter, American College Health Association, 46*(1).
2. 45 CFR 160.103. Standards for Privacy of Individually Identifiable Health Information. US Department of Health and Human Services, Office for Civil Rights. (2000, December 28).
3. 45 CFR 164.520(b)(3). Health Insurance Reform: Security Standards, Final Rule. US Department of Health and Human Services, Office for Civil Rights. (2003, February 20).

Chapter 3

The Family and Medical Leave Act (FMLA): Making Managing More Humane But More Difficult

Kendall Cortelyou-Ward, PhD, *Program Director, MS-Healthcare Informatics, Department of Health Management and Informatics, College of Health and Public Affairs, University of Central Florida, Orlando, Florida*

Andrea Velez-Vazquez, MS, *Academic Coordinator, Human Resource Management, Department of Health Management and Informatics, College of Health and Public Affairs, University of Central Florida, Orlando, Florida*

Timothy Rotarius, PhD, MBA, *Professor & Vice Chair, Department of Health Management and Informatics, College of Health and Public Affairs, University of Central Florida, Orlando, Florida*

Chapter Objectives

- Briefly trace the evolution of the Family and Medical Leave Act (FMLA) and examine the reasons for its eventual passage in 1993, including a review of related legislation.
- Understand the rules governing applicability of and eligibility for employee leave under FMLA as well as the FMLA requirements placed on employers.
- Describe and define the various forms of leave available under FMLA.
- Review some pertinent legal cases involving FMLA and note what was learned from them.
- Examine the managerial implications of FMLA in terms of its effects on staffing and scheduling and the costs of operating.

Introduction

The US healthcare industry operates in a hyperturbulent environment. Organizations must contend with a barrage of competing and conflicting environmental factors that involve such current concerns as professional caregiver shortages, dwindling reimbursements, malpractice concerns, accreditation issues, and government regulations. This chapter examines the organizational issues associated with one specific government regulation, the Family and Medical Leave Act (FMLA).

The FMLA became law in 1993. According to the FMLA website (http://www.dol.gov/esa/whd/fmla), this act requires a covered employer to grant an eligible employee up to a total of 12 workweeks of unpaid leave during any 12-month period for one or more of the following reasons: the birth and care of the newborn child of the employee; placement with the employee of a son or daughter for adoption or foster care; the need to care for an immediate family member (spouse, child, or parent) with a serious health condition; or personally take medical leave when the employee is unable to work because of a serious health condition.

This chapter will examine the FMLA from its beginnings in discussions to its fruition as federal legislation. Next, FMLA eligibility and types of FMLA leave will be presented. This will be followed by a discussion of issues of concern to healthcare managers.

Background

The FMLA of 1993 represented the culmination of intense debate in the US Congress beginning during the 1950s. Throughout the decades since FMLA's concepts were first introduced into the public discussion, both public perception of the need for FMLA and business perspective of the value of FMLA have changed.

Initially, both the public and the business community rejected the concepts in today's FMLA. Then the public came to realize the importance of FMLA's concepts as applied to balancing work life with personal life. Businesses soon followed suit and also began to recognize the importance of FMLA's concepts.

History of Legislation

The FMLA has an interesting history that goes back to the 1950s when Congress began holding discussions on issues related to women in the workplace. This led to several proposed pieces of legislations, some of which were voted into law and some that never made it through the legislative process. These myriad activities eventually resulted in passage of the FMLA in 1993. The congressional discussions of the 1950s focused mainly on gender discrimination. According to Dehan, this was because women were usually their family's primary caretakers.[1] Women represented almost half of the workforce and were still expected to fulfill their familial obligations as well. Working women were often discriminated against in the workplace. Few states regulated leave policies, so organizations had free reign to take whatever action they wished; this often resulted in job loss for women.

Thousands of families across the country were faced with issues that required women to choose between their families and jobs. In an effort to remedy this issue of state of affairs, congressional advocates felt compelled to pass legislation to allow women to take leave from their jobs for an extended period to handle family matters.

Pregnancy Discrimination Act

In the 1970s, President Carter's administration developed a plan to address the critical issue of pregnancy of employed women. The Pregnancy Discrimination Act (PDA) became law in October 1978, amending Title VII of the Civil Rights Act of 1964. The PDA made illegal the discrimination arising in response to childbirth, medical conditions associated with childbirth, and maternity care. It required companies to treat disabilities associated with childbirth as any other disability.[2] Those who supported and advocated for PDA acknowledged, however, that PDA did not grant special privileges. Instead, PDA addressed an individual's civil rights and thus resulted in increased support for gender equality.[3]

Child Care Act

The proposed Child Care Act of 1979 was intended to provide child care options to parents and provide school-based child care programs. The provisions dealing with child care options available to parents cover similar territory as some of the provisions found in the final FMLA legislation. However, the bill lacked congressional support because constituents of various teaching and educational interest groups held conflicting views, which resulted in failure to form a successful coalition.[4]

Parental and Disability Act

In 1985, Congresswoman Patricia Schroeder of Colorado introduced into Congress the Parental and Disability Act. This proposed legislation was to provide employees with 18 weeks of unpaid leave for birth, child adoption, serious child illnesses, and disabilities. This bill received immediate resistance from businesses; according to their estimates the legislation would cost commerce approximately $16 billion annually. The bill was considered not financially feasible.[5]

For 7 years, Representative Schroeder continued to introduce the same bill to Congress. During that time it was revised numerous times with the intention of meeting employee needs by providing a reasonable amount of time to handle family affairs while preventing major disruptions in the workplace. A major US Supreme Court decision in 1987 affected the content of the bill. In this particular case, the justices upheld a decree and stated that parental leave should be granted to all workers and should not be limited to women only.[6]

Family and Medical Leave Act of 1993

After additional amendments were introduced into the Parental and Disability Act, the act was ultimately renamed, becoming known as the FMLA. This legislation was signed into law in February 1993 by President Clinton and went into effect in August 1993. The FMLA remains a fluid act, ready to adapt to new situations. For example, in 2008, FMLA was expanded to cover various situations unique to military families. The US Department of Labor issued guidelines in January 2009 regarding how to handle individuals affected by these specific military situations.

Practical Considerations

The realization of the need for legislation such as FMLA was in direct response to gender discrimination and work-life balance issues facing the American workforce. Prior to the passage of FMLA, few organizations offered family leave benefits. Employees who were not eligible for benefits were either forced to leave their jobs or seek alternative means to fulfill family obligations. Unfortunately, many families did not have the option of having the mother stay home to focus on family matters since approximately one third of a family's income was earned by a woman and the loss of a household income created a large financial burden.[7] Women who left their jobs to assume the role as the unemployed primary caretaker saw their lifestyles change significantly because their households had to adjust to surviving on one income.

Over time, the federal government received sufficient feedback from the public to indicate that it was necessary to address the crisis nationwide. The FMLA provided a solution to enable working families to provide care and attention to family affairs without the risk of losing their jobs.

Why, however, did it take 40 years of discussion to finally arrive at the passage of the FMLA? Initially, there was a lack of public support for legislation covering the familial rights of women in the workplace. During the many years of stakeholder and congressional discussion, there were often inconsistent and competing claims from activist groups. In addition, businesses, which were heavy political contributors, were often vocal about the perceived productivity drop and enhanced dollar costs of involved in providing this type of employee benefit.

How were these obstacles overcome? It is likely that the sheer magnitude of women in the workforce, plus the recognized upward career mobility of women, contributed to the ultimate passing of federal legislation. For example, during the 40 years from the 1950s to the 1990s, the amount of women in the American work-force increased by approximately 47%.[7] In addition, during this same era, women began assuming higher and higher levels of responsibility in businesses.

Types of Leave and Eligibility Criteria

The FMLA is an entitlement like federal law. This means that if certain criteria are met, an employee is entitled to coverage by the specific guidelines and rules.

Organizational Applicability

According to the article "Providing Notice to Employees on Leave," approximately 42% of America's workforce is not entitled to FMLA leave.[8] The FMLA extends coverage to federal employees and to private organizations having 50 or more employees within 75 miles of the work location for at least 20 weeks of the year.[2] Consequently, organizations that do not meet the set criteria are not required to extend FMLA benefits to their employees.

For employees to receive FMLA benefits, they must be employed with a covered organization for a minimum of 12 months and must have worked a minimum of 1250 hours within the year.[2] Individuals who meet these requirements are eligible (but not required) to request FMLA leave. An employee who has a foreseeable circumstance, such as pregnancy, must provide at least 30 days notice. Employees are required to provide supporting documentation when requesting leave and the employer can request additional documentation to substantiate the leave request.[9] A request may be denied if the employee does not provide this required notice. It is extremely important for organizations to follow the prescribed protocol to prevent complications that can escalate to legal complaints.

Organizations are mandated by the federal government to notify employees of FMLA provisions by placing an informational poster in a conspicuous area. The purpose of posting this information is to ensure employee awareness of the act and to facilitate employee review of the provisions outlined in the act.

Employee Eligibility

The FMLA is intended to provide a sense of work-life balance to working families by offering eligible employees 12 weeks of unpaid leave to focus on family or health issues while also maintaining job protection. Leave requirements have evolved since the act was originally passed and not only cover women but also provide equal family rights to men as well. Although women usually take maternity leave to care for a newborn or ill child, fathers can also exercise their rights and take time to dedicate to family affairs with all the protections afforded by the act.

Certain employees can be exempt from FMLA assistance. Some key employees (defined as those who earn in the top 10% of salaries for the firm) may be exempt from FMLA leave if the company demonstrates that the employee's absence causes serious economic damage to the organization.[10]

Employees who are eligible for FMLA can utilize paid time off or take unpaid leave if paid leave is not available.[10] During the leave period, employers are mandated by the federal government to continue offering all benefits to which the employee would be entitled under normal circumstances. This includes medical benefits—health insurance coverage must be offered continuously to all members in the plan while on FMLA leave.[10] After the expiration of a leave, an employee must be returned to his or her original position, or to an equivalent position.[11]

The act has several detailed provisions that control how employees take leave and the manner in which organizations must manage the process. The law provides employees with two types of leave: (1) 12 continuous weeks of unpaid leave and (2) intermittent leave or a modified work schedule.

Type of Leave: 12 Weeks of Unpaid Leave

Section 102 of FMLA indicates that eligible employees are entitled to 12 weeks of unpaid leave for the following reasons: (a) birth and care for a newborn child; (b) adoption of a child or placement of a foster child; (c) care for an immediate family member (spouse, child, or parent) who has a serious medical condition; or (d) a serious medical condition of the employee that prevents him or her from performing normal job duties. In addition, in 2008, the following eligibility reason was added: (e) if an employee's spouse, child, or parent is on active duty or call-to-active-duty status as a member of the National Guard or Reserves in support of a contingency operation.[12]

Before FMLA was enacted, Congress debated the amount of leave time an employee would require to handle family affairs while ensuring minimal adverse impact on the employer. It was finally decided that 12 weeks was reasonable for both employee and organization. Court cases have since determined that, during an employee's absence, the organization has the right to make certain limited operating adjustments to facilitate the proper conduct of business operations when an employee exercises his or her FMLA rights.

Type of Leave: Intermittent Leave or Modified Work Schedules

Intermittent leave and modified work schedules are extended to employees who have serious medical conditions or have immediate family members experiencing serious medical conditions.[13] According to FMLA's provisions, "A serious health condition is defined as an illness, injury, impairment, or physical or mental condition that involves inpatient care in a hospital, hospice or residential medical care facility, or continuing treatment by a health care provider."[8]

The conditions of this type of leave require that leave is deemed to be "medically necessary" to attend medical appointments or seek medical treatment associated with a medical condition.[13] Employees who demonstrate difficulty fulfilling their responsibilities as a result of their medical condition are eligible to receive accommodations set forth by the employer. The employee can be placed in an alternative position with the same rate of pay and unchanged benefits. Employers who extend this benefit will be in compliance with FMLA's Intermittent Leave Policies and the American Disabilities Act.[13]

Summary of Eligibility and Leave

The organizational and employee eligibility criteria and the two types of FMLA leave presented here are simply brief summaries of a complex piece of legislation. Organizations usually entrust the oversight of compliance with FMLA provisions to the organization's HR department. However, FMLA significantly affects the operational side of the organization. For example, managers almost always face staffing concerns when employees utilize the FMLA benefit. In addition, FMLA provisions do not waive or supersede other federal and state labor relations laws or union collective bargaining agreements.

Selected Legal Cases Pertaining to FMLA

Over the years, there have been numerous lawsuits centering about alleged violations of FMLA rights. It is imperative that both employees and employers fully understand the provisions of FMLA in an effort to reduce the chance of any particular situation moving into the judicial system. Two cases, *Ragsdale v. Wolverine Worldwide, Inc.* and *Nevada Department of Human Resources v. William Hibbs* address the ways in which employees and organizations are impacted when FMLA provisions are misinterpreted.

Ragsdale v. Wolverine Worldwide, Inc.

This case involved Tracy Ragsdale and her employer, Wolverine Worldwide, Inc. Ragsdale had been employed by Wolverine Worldwide for 11 months, during which time she was diagnosed with Hodgkin's disease.[14] Subsequently, Ragsdale was told by her medical provider that her medical condition would require intense treatment that would render her unable to work. Ragsdale relayed this information to her employer. Wolverine Worldwide subsequently informed Ragsdale that since she had been employed for less than 1 year, she was not entitled to FMLA benefits.

Wolverine Worldwide, however, had a generous internal medical leave policy. Ragsdale was informed that she was entitled to medical leave per Wolverine Worldwide's company leave policy. This policy provided employees up to 30 weeks of unpaid sick leave, approximately a 7-month period. Per Wolverine Worldwide's human resources policy guidelines, during the benefit coverage period, Ragsdale would be required to request extensions every 30 days. Ragsdale applied for this company medical leave and took her first 30 days of leave. Ragsdale subsequently requested 30 day extensions for 7 months of allowable coverage.

Wolverine Worldwide continuously granted Ragsdale's leave requests throughout the 7-month time period. At the end of the period, Wolverine Worldwide denied Ragsdale's request for another 30-day extension. At this particular time, after seeking clearance from her physician, Ragsdale requested a modified work schedule. Wolverine Worldwide subsequently denied Ragsdale's request for a modified work schedule.

Next, Ragsdale requested FMLA leave because, counting her 7 months of unpaid medical leave, she had now been employed with the organization for longer than 1 year. Wolverine Worldwide denied her request for FMLA. Subsequently, Ragsdale was terminated by Wolverine Worldwide because she had exhausted all of her paid and unpaid leave (per the company's leave policy) and because she abandoned her job by not returning to work.

Ragsdale filed a lawsuit in the US District Court for the Eastern District of Arkansas claiming that she was entitled to 12 additional weeks of medical leave under FMLA. During the discovery portion of the case, Ragsdale learned that 12 weeks of the medical leave she used had been classified by Wolverine Worldwide as FMLA leave.

Ragsdale's legal arguments claimed that since the employer had not told her that 12 weeks of medical leave had been classified as FMLA leave, Ragsdale was still entitled to the FMLA leave. The District Court of Arkansas ruled that Ragsdale was indeed entitled to 12 additional weeks of FMLA after she reached her 1-year anniversary; however, the court issued summary judgment to Wolverine Worldwide indicating that Ragsdale used faulty substantiation of her claim, which rendered her claim invalid.[15]

Ragsdale filed an appeal to the Eighth Circuit Court of Appeals, which found that entitlement of FMLA cannot start until an employee is notified by the employer. However, this appeals court also found Ragsdale's claim to be invalid.[15] The case ended up in the US Supreme Court. The justices averted the central issue concerning whether or not Ragsdale was entitled to 12 weeks of FMLA leave and instead emphasized the monetary penalties assessed to organizations that fail to provide adequate FMLA notification to their employees.

This case highlighted several factors that affect employers. First, employers need to be specific about the process used to inform employees about their FMLA rights. In addition, although it is compassionate and generous for companies to provide more than 12 weeks of medical leave, organizations must consider the future ramifications involved when providing extended leave policies. Misinterpretation or lack of information can adversely impact employers.

Nevada Department of Human Resources v. William Hibbs

This case focuses on gender discrimination in the state of Nevada's leave policies. In 1997, William Hibbs was employed by the Nevada Department of Human

Resources. Hibbs, who was eligible for FMLA benefits, requested FMLA leave to care for his ill wife. Hibbs was granted and used 12 weeks of leave. After utilizing all of his FMLA leave time, Hibbs did not comply with his company's request that he return to work. Hibbs was subsequently terminated for job abandonment.

Hibbs filed suit against the Nevada Department of Human Resources in the US District Court District of Nevada alleging that his FMLA rights were violated. After review, the District Court ruled in Nevada's favor, indicating that the state was provided immunity under the Eleventh Amendment. Hibbs then appealed the lower court's decision because he felt he was entitled to more leave time and also alleged that he was discriminated against because of his gender. Subsequently, the Ninth Court of Appeals effectively removed Nevada's immunity from Section 5 of FMLA.[16]

According to Kulig, Section 5 of FMLA was intended to provide parameters to the Eleventh Amendment by bestowing upon Congress the ability to impose stipulations such as equal protection of the Fourteenth Amendment.[16] Section 5 says that states that use gender to evaluate FMLA claims are subject to scrutiny tests to determine the constitutionality of this evaluation method. These tests are known as congruence and proportionality tests and are used to examine the constitutionality or unconstitutionality of a state's conduct. After the state of Nevada underwent these tests, the US Supreme Court ruled that Nevada acted in an unconstitutional manner based on gender discrimination inherent in the state's leave policies.[16]

The US Supreme Court sided with the Eighth Circuit Court of Appeals when it ruled that states do not possess immunity and must, therefore, comply with FMLA provisions. In other words, individual states must abide by federal regulations since states are not summarily exempted from the rule. The US Supreme Court stated that although the Eleventh Amendment indicates states are granted immunity and cannot be sued, the Fourteenth Amendment provides the US Supreme Court the power to compel states to follow federal policies.

Summary of Legal Cases

The two foregoing cases provide insight into the complexity of FMLA-related issues. Case law regarding the interpretation of FMLA sets precedents concerning about how organizations integrate FMLA into their human resources policies. Workplace issues such as those discussed in these two cases provide but a small sample of the breadth of workplace issues that can and do arise in the healthcare industry.

Managerial Implications

Leave policies under the FMLA hold implications for management in four particular areas of concern: (a) staff planning and the use of FMLA; (b) financial implications of FMLA; (c) employee morale and use of FMLA; and (d) fraud and abuse of FMLA.

Staff Planning and the Use of FMLA

One of the biggest challenges that accompany the FMLA is planning for employees who will be on medical leave either intermittently or for extended periods of time. In health care, where personnel shortages are sometimes commonplace, there is a heightened focus on staffing requirements. While even the most well-prepared manager can find this focus on properly staffing the facility to be a daunting challenge, managers must ensure that their departments can continue to function regardless of who may be out on leave. Various tools exist to facilitate staff planning when employees utilize FMLA benefits. Two of these tools are cross training current employees and employing agency workers.

Cross Training

Cross training is the process of training employees to work in areas other than their regularly scheduled assignments. Cross training can be an effective way to plan for staff absences and to also ensure proper allocation of resources. The use of cross training is especially effective when employees take intermittent family or medical leave. The process of cross training varies greatly between clinical and nonclinical workers and thus should be considered to involve two distinct procedures.

Cross Training Clinical Employees.   The use of cross training in nursing has been the subject of considerable discussion throughout the literature.[17,18] By training nurses to work on different floors and also across different clinical and functional departments, healthcare managers can reduce reliance on agency or temporary workers while seeking to preserve budgetary resources. Also, cross-trained nurses can experience enhanced career fulfillment by expanding their skill sets. When managers formally incorporate cross-training processes into a healthcare firm's staffing plan, managers can easily call upon nurses already employed, trained, and vetted by the organization to step in when an employee takes intermittent family medical leave.

Cross Training Nonclinical Employees.   Cross training nonclinical employees can be more problematic than cross-departmental training for clinical employees such as nurses. In addition, in the actual process of cross training nonclinical employees, cross training can be especially difficult in the case of managers and supervisors who take FMLA leave. Nonclinical employees already tend to be involved in a wide range of day-to-day activities, the subtleties of which may be difficult for a substitute employee to completely grasp.

For example, an administrative assistant in marketing would conceivably have significantly different duties from an administrative assistant in human resources. In such cases, it can prove to be quite challenging to pursue cross training of administrative personnel. In cases such as these, managers might find it more effective to cross train within the department rather than cross training between departments.

Agency Workers

Temporary or agency workers are not directly employed by the organization that uses their services. Instead, these workers are actually employees of a staffing agency that contracts with, for example, the hospital to provide nursing staff.[19] Agency workers can be used to cover either intermittent or long-term leave and have been historically relied upon extensively by healthcare organizations. Again, depending on the type of organization and the type of employee taking leave (i.e., clinical versus nonclinical), agency workers may or may not be the best solution for family-leave–related absences.

Clinical Agency Workers. The use of agency nurses in healthcare organizations (particularly hospitals) has been hotly debated in the literature for many years.[20] Negative issues that can arise when utilizing agency nurses include possible lower quality of care provided, increased malpractice exposure, lack of continuity of care, and significantly higher personnel costs. While it is unlikely that all of these potential problems apply in every agency situation, managers would be well advised to include these factors in any analysis prior to utilizing clinical agency workers.

All potential negative outcomes aside, given the actual high utilization of agency nurses, it appears that agency clinicians are a valuable resource for healthcare managers. Assuming that the possible negatives can be eliminated or controlled, agency nurses are especially valuable for managers confronted with employees taking extended family or medical leave. For example, when an employee has a child and takes off the maximum 12 weeks of parental leave, finding cross-trained employees to cover each shift will likely produce an overall frustrated and frazzled staff. Rather, a manager will often find it more conducive to a positive work environment to hire an agency nurse to cover the entire 12 weeks of medical leave. This would result in minimal disruption of the normal work flow as experienced by the regular employees.

Nonclinical Employees. Much like clinical agency workers, nonclinical agency workers can be a suitable fill-in for nonclinical employees taking extended family medical leave. Given the diverse nature and specialized knowledge required by many nonclinical employees, managers likely would find that bringing in competent, functionally skilled, nonclinical agency replacements will provide the best continuity for day-to-day operations.

Financial Implications of the FMLA

Regardless of the method used to accommodate a leave mandated by the FMLA, there are certain inherent financial implications to be addressed. For example, even though the leave taken under FMLA is unpaid, employers are still responsible for accrued employee benefits, including healthcare benefits, to which the employee is entitled.

Even though theoretically, the absent employee is no longer paid by the organization, the cost of benefits, which can run 30% or more of an employee's salary, can present a tremendous financial burden on the healthcare organization.[21] Additional financial obligations can be incurred by the use of agency workers and training costs.

Agency Workers

A major disadvantage in the use of agency workers is the associated cost. For example, because the healthcare facility does not hire an agency nurse directly, there is usually an added fee that is paid directly to the staffing agency. This "retainer like" fee is inherent in the use of agency nurses. This fee varies greatly depending on the type of nurse employed and the duration of the contracts between the agency worker and the staffing agency and between the healthcare firm and the staffing agency. Over time, these fees can present a significant cost to the healthcare organization.

Training Costs

Training costs are necessarily incurred to prepare employees whether by straight-forward training or specific job orientation. Training costs are incurred in a variety of situations: when an organization hires a new employee; when a firm cross trains current employees; or when an organization contracts with an agency for temporary employees. Also, it is important for managers to consider accreditation requirements when planning a training schedule. Thus, training costs associated with the use of family medical leave can vary greatly depending on the type of employee, the skill sets required of the employee, and the mechanism used to replace this employee's on-the-job task performance.

Employee Morale and Use of the FMLA

Employee morale is an extremely important consideration in the acceptance of and adherence to any policy or procedure enacted in the workplace. When an employee takes family or medical leave, the issue of morale becomes increasingly important as other workers can feel "put upon" by the absent worker. Whether an organization uses agency workers, cross training, or simply asks current employees to fill-in for the missing employee, there is no question that the morale of the organization can suffer from FMLA-related absences.

Morale and the Use of Agency Workers

Bringing agency workers into the organization can have varying effects on the morale of the employees who are already there. A study of hospital nurse managers revealed that managers perceive a lower status associated with graduate nurses who pursue agency work directly out of college, but these same managers perceive a greater respect for experienced nurses who choose to work as agency employees.[22] These differences in perception can and do affect the morale of both other employees and less experienced agency nurses.

Morale and the Use of Cross Training

Cross training generally has a positive effect on employee morale. For example, many employees see the opportunity to learn additional skills as a positive experience that helps them to grow in both their skills and their profession.[17] However, cross training can also have a profoundly negative effect on morale as well. If employees are forced to cross train and are not appropriately compensated or recognized for the additional skills sets acquired via cross training, the burden of cross training can have negative effects on already overworked staff.

Fraud and Abuse of the FMLA

The FMLA, like other entitlement programs, possesses considerable potential for abuse. Organizational policy is often not sufficient to prevent abuses; however, there are steps managers and organizations can take to minimize the possibility of FMLA "fraud and abuse" such as requiring fitness-for-duty certification, requiring recertification of the underlying medical condition, and establishing uniform policies.

Requiring Fitness for Duty Certification

If FMLA leave was taken for an employee's own personal health reasons and if required by the organization's policy, an employer can require an employee to submit certification from a physician that he or she is indeed healthy enough to return to work at the conclusion of the leave.[23] This fitness-for-duty certification need only be a short letter from a healthcare professional but can provide tremendous support for the organization in the event of an FMLA-related lawsuit.

Requiring Recertification of Medical Condition

Using the standard of "reasonable basis," an employer can request that an employee utilizing FMLA leave periodically secure a recertification of his or her medical condition. This most often applies when an employee is using intermittent FMLA leave for a chronic condition. The definition of "reasonable basis" varies depending on the situation but is often interpreted to mean no more often than once every 30 days. However, if an employer suspects FMLA fraud based upon a clear pattern of abuse, employers can request recertification more often. One example of possible FMLA abuse is evident when an employee displays a pattern of Monday or Friday absences that are supposedly FMLA related. The manager would be well advised to request recertification more often than every 30 days under such circumstances.

Establishing Uniform Policies

Establishing and publicizing appropriate policies and enforcing them uniformly is essential to any well-run organization. This can be especially relevant when dealing with medical leave requests. It is essential that organizations treat all employees the same regardless of status or hierarchic level. Two policies that can help combat FMLA abuse address call-in procedures and secondary employment.

Many organizations require employees to call in to a manager within a certain timeframe if they are going to be absent from work. This call-in procedure is generally uniform across the organization, with repercussions specified for those employees deviating from policy and not abiding by the rules. Absences related to FMLA leave should be subject to the same standards as sick leave taken by other employees. This policy should be put in place and communicated to employees before FMLA leave is granted. The second suggested policy, addressing secondary employment, should exist simply to advise employees that working for another employer while on FMLA leave constitutes abuse of the conditions of the FMLA.

Summary of Managerial Implications

Encountering FMLA-related absences has become a way of life for all managers, especially managers in the stressful world of healthcare delivery. When employees avail themselves of the federally mandated FMLA leave, managers need to ensure (a) that their departments are adequately staffed; (b) that their budgets include sufficient funds for both cross-training opportunities as well as for hiring agency workers; (c) that overall employee morale is not adversely affected by employees on FMLA leave; and that employees are not abusing the FMLA benefit.

Conclusion

The FMLA of 1993 was the culmination of 40 years of congressional debate. The FMLA provides generous benefits to employees who experience health-related family situations that require their full attention. As such, FMLA is a compassionate measure that seeks to provide a level of comfort to employees so that the employee can deal with the crisis while being assured that the employee will still have a job and the associated pay and benefits once the medical crisis has passed.

Managers should see the FMLA and tangentially related legislation as opportunities to reach out to employees and say, "We are here for you." While this federal law places some burdens on employers, the burdens are not designed or expected to be onerous to any organization. Managers need to comply with the rules of FMLA, while always being on the lookout for those few instances of fraud and abuse. The organization's official policies should reflect recognition of the importance of the FMLA to a strong and productive workforce.

Questions for Review and Discussion

1. In your best judgment, why did it take some 40 years to finally arrive at the passage of the FMLA?
2. In what ways has FMLA bettered the circumstances of workers?
3. What must then occur if an employee's job is necessarily filled permanently while he or she is on leave under FMLA?
4. Are all employees eligible for leave under FMLA? If not, why might there be differences?
5. What significant piece of legislation was replaced by FMLA, and how does FMLA differ from its predecessor?
6. In what ways might FMLA have made managing a department more difficult?
7. Of all of its conditions and requirements, what do you believe is the single, principal reason for FMLA's existence?
8. In what ways may managers react to the staffing and scheduling difficulties that may accompany some FMLA leaves?
9. Why is it recommended that the organization have uniform policies for application of FMLA?
10. What recourses were available before the passage of FMLA to employees in need of extended time off?

References

1. Dehan, P. (2002). Has the FMLA been stretched beyond its intended scope? *Northern Kentuckey Law Review, 29*(3), 629–640.
2. Ruhm, C. (1997). Policy watch: The Family and Medical Leave Act. *Journal of Economic Perspectives, 11*(3), 175–186.
3. Zigler, E., & Meryl, F. (1988). *The parental leave crisis: Toward a national policy.* New Haven, CT: Yale University Press.
4. Wisensale, S. (1997). The White House and Congress on child care and family leave policy—From Carter to Clinton. *Policy Studies Journal, 25*(1), 75–86.

5. Selmi, M. (2004). Is something better than nothing? Critical reflections on ten years of the FMLA. *Journal of Law and Policy, 15*(65), 65–90.

6. Radigan, A. (1988). The evolution of family leave legislation in the U.S. Congress. Women's research and education paper. Washington, DC: Women's Research and Education Institute.

7. Caputo, R. (2000). Race and marital history as correlates of women's access to family-friendly employee benefits. *Journal of Family and Economic Issues, 21*(4), 365–385.

8. Cossi, P., & McGovern, D. (2003). Providing notice to employees on leave—Implications of Ragsdale v. Wolverine Worlwide, Inc. *American Association of Occupational Health Nurses Journal, 51*(11), 8.

9. Morris, J. (2008). Integrated absence management and the Family and Medical Leave Act. *American Association of Occupational Health Nurses Journal, 56*(5), 207–216.

10. Lewison, J. (1993). Family and medical leave becomes a bill. *Journal of Accountacy, 175*(5), 22–23.

11. Bank, M., & Hitchings, T. E. (1994). *Facts on file yearbook 1993*. New York, NY: Infobase Holdings.

12. US Department of Labor. (2009). Wage and hour division: Family and Medical Leave Act. Available at: http://www.dol.gov/whd/fmla/index.htm. Accessed May 21, 2010.

13. Fernstrom, S., & Pranschke, S. (1993). Labor Department regulations for Family and Medical Leave Act. *Benefits Quarterly, 9*(4).

14. Hesse, K. (2003). FMLA–notice. *Benefits Quarterly, 19*(2), 104.

15. Brown, J., Mero, N., & Robinson, R. (2003). Employer penalties for failure to provide employee notification under the Family and Medical Leave Act: "Clarifications" following Ragsdale v. Wolverine Worldwide, Inc. *Employee Responsibilites and Rights Journal, 15*(1), 11.

16. Kulig, G. (2004). Constitutional law—The Family and Medical Leave Act: Abrogation of states' immunity from suit—Nevada Department of Human Resources v. Hibbs, 538 U.S. 721. *Suffolk University Law Review, 38*(1), 231–237.

17. Inman, R., Blumenfeld, B., & Ko, A. (2005). Cross training nurses to reduce staffing costs. *Health Care Management Review, 30*(2), 116–125.

18. Gnanlet, A., & Gilland, W. (2009). Sequential and simultaneous decision making for optimizing health care resource flexibilities. *Decision Sciences, 40*(2), 295–326.

19. Bloom, A., Alexander, J. A., & Nuchols, B. A. (1997). Nursing staff patterns and hospital efficiency in the United States. *Social Sciences and Medicine, 44*(2), 147–155.

20. Needleman, J., Buerhaus, J., Mattke, S., Stewart, M., & Zelevinksy, K. (2002). Nursing staffing levels and the quality of care in hospitals. *New England Journal of Medicine, 346*(22), 1715–1722.

21. US Bureau of Labor Statistics. (2009). *Employer costs for employee compensation summary*. Available at: www.bls.gov. Accessed October 13, 2009.

22. Manias, E., Aitken, R., Peerson, A., Parker, J., & Wong, K. (2003). Agency nursing work in acute care settings—Perceptions of hospital nursing managers and agency nurse providers. *Journal of Clinical Nursing, 12*(4), 457–466.

23. US Department of Labor. (2009). *Fitness for duty certification*. Available at: http://www.dol.gov/dol/allcfr/title_29/Part_825/29CFR825.312.htm. Accessed on May 21, 2010.

Chapter 4

The Americans with Disabilities Act (ADA): How "Reasonable" Is Reasonable Accommodation?

Sandra K. Collins, MBA, ABD, *Assistant Professor, School of Allied Health, Southern Illinois University–Carbondale, Carbondale, Illinois*

Chapter Objectives

- Introduce the Americans with Disabilities Act (ADA) as an important civil rights statute and review its evolution from earlier legislation through the Civil Rights Act of 1964 and the Rehabilitation Act of 1973, and address the significant effects of the ADA amendments of 2008.
- Develop an understanding of "disability" as describing various physical and mental impairments and an appreciation of the fact that there is not always a precise definition available.
- Describe in general those kinds of impairments that are legitimately considered disabilities, as well as providing examples of sometimes-disputed conditions that are not legitimate disabilities.
- Define "essential job functions" as applied to potential employment for impaired individuals, and define "reasonable accommodation" and the attendant responsibilities of management.
- Review a number of examples of cases necessitating legal determination of whether a particular condition did or did not constitute a disability.

Introduction

The Americans with Disabilities Act (ADA) is a complex piece of legislation that perplexes managers from every business sector. Complex legal terms such as reasonable accommodation, undue hardship, major life activities, and essential job functions complicate the interpretation of the guidelines provided in this significant civil rights statute.

Written to protect employable individuals with disabilities, the ADA has been through a number of changes since its inception. Even cursory study will reveal that an increase in the number of cases that allege disability discrimination may be on the rise.[1] This presents healthcare managers with an ever-changing challenge in terms of developing ongoing ways by which to offer disabled workers equal employment opportunities and protecting their organizations from costly legal ramifications.

History and Evolution

The Civil Rights Act of 1964, specifically the part known as Title VII, provided the legal foundation by which all people were permitted to pursue any type of work they desired without discrimination based on race, color, religion, gender, or national origin. Restrictions placed on individuals could only be those that were self-imposed and based on their qualifications, talents, energies, and desires. Title VII specifically prohibited creating discriminatory limits and segregating or classifying employees or job applicants in ways that robbed them from equal employment opportunities.

The Equal Employment Opportunity Commission (EEOC) emerged from the mandates brought forth in Title VII. This group was charged with the responsibility of enforcing the antidiscrimination regulations set forth in the Civil Rights Act. Although individuals with disabilities were initially mentioned in the Title VII legislation, they were more specifically addressed in the Rehabilitation Act of 1973. The Rehabilitation Act recognized and addressed the multitude of myths and biases associated with employing disabled workers, and legislators sought to apply more rigid guidelines and consequences for employers who attempted to discriminate against those with disabilities.[1]

Spurred by 120,000 soldiers returning from war with permanent disabilities, the Rehabilitation Act of 1973 emerged and addressed disability discrimination.[2] However, the mandates included in this legislation at this time applied only to federal government employees and employers conducting a certain amount of business with the government.[1] Therefore, further amendments to Title VII were deemed necessary and were introduced in 1990 through the ADA.

The ADA is a significant civil rights statute specifically covering individuals with disabilities. Written and overseen by the EEOC, the ADA prohibits employers from discriminating against qualified individuals with disabilities with regard to all employment transactions.[3] Initially, it applied to private-sector employers and departments or agencies of state or local government that employed 25 or more persons. In 1994, the act was revised and remained applicable to those same employers but the number of employees was reduced to 15 or more.[4] The ADA was amended again in 2008, making some significant changes in definitions and conditions governing the applicability of portions of the act.

The 2008 amendments provided a mandate to the EEOC to issue binding regulations and other guidance to further clarify the law. The Supreme Court had questioned the EEOC's rule-making authority under the original ADA; the amendments firmly establish the EEOC's authority.

The ADA provides the same protection that is given to minorities and other protected groups outlined in the Civil Rights Act of 1964.[5] Included in the protective mechanisms of ADA are all employment transactions such as job applications, hiring, discharge, compensation, promotion, training, or other terms, conditions, or privileges of employment. The ADA also sets forth guidelines that indicate that employers are required to make reasonable accommodations for the physical and mental limitations of their employees unless doing so causes an undue hardship on the business.[6, 7]

In order to appropriately address the numerous complexities associated with ADA issues, healthcare managers need to examine policies either currently in use or in need of implementation. This introspective effort may require extensive evaluation of the organizational processes associated with recruitment, application forms, position descriptions, interviewing and selection, employee testing, compensation policies, performance standards, and the training, evaluation, promotion, discipline, and termination of employees.[8]

The most common criticism often given regarding the ADA involves the lack of specificity. Although the ADA is cited as being a major civil rights statute, it is rather elusive in terms of precise rules or guidance for employers. Cases are reviewed on a case-by-case basis and the elusiveness of the approach seemingly was the EEOC's original intent. They reportedly thought that the case-by-case approach was essential in terms of assuring that qualified individuals with varying abilities were given an equal opportunity to vie for a wide variety of jobs. However, the lack of specificity makes it difficult for employers to know exactly how to comply with ADA regulations. Instead of precise guidance, the ADA only provides parameters to aid employers in how to consider disabling conditions in terms of employment.[3]

Defining and Identifying Disability

Negative stigmas associated with the disabled, especially those in the mental realm, were cultivated and developed many decades ago. Prior to World War II, many individuals born with a disability faced a life of institutionalization and were afforded few benefits associated with their constitutional right to pursue happiness. Eugenicists amplified the negative persona associated with the disabled when they began supporting laws prohibiting the mentally disabled from marrying. Since some eugenicists went as far as to promote mandatory sterilization of those considered biologically inadequate, it is not difficult to establish that many prejudices and discriminatory practices emerged from the foundational beliefs cultivated in earlier years.[9,10]

The intention behind the development of the ADA was to amplify the employment potential of individuals with disabilities.[7] The term disability is loosely defined within ADA legislation, but includes not only physical limitations, but hearing and visual impairments, paraplegia, epilepsy, HIV or AIDS, and many other conditions.

One effect of the 2008 amendments was to instruct employers as well as the courts to adopt a broad standard in determining whether an individual may be considered disabled, providing a greater scope of protection for employees. This action essentially reverses years of conservative court decisions and in effect ensures that more ADA cases will go to trial rather than being dismissed at earlier stages.

Although somewhat elusive and vague, there are three general guidelines provided by the ADA, which offer guidance in defining a disability. These include the following:

1. A physical or mental impairment (such as epilepsy, blindness, deafness, or paralysis), which significantly limits one or more major life activities (caring for oneself, performing manuals tasks, walking, running, seeing, hearing, speaking, breathing, learning, thinking, sitting, standing, reaching, lifting, concentrating, sleeping, or interacting with others.[7,11]

2. A verifiable record of the impairment is available. This may include individuals having a history of a disability such as cancer, heart disease, or mental disorder.[7]

3. Indications that the individual is regarded as having an impairment. This would include those impairments that do not necessarily limit a major life activity but are predetermined by the ADA as impairments that are accentuated by the attitudes of others. For example, an individual disfigured from a fire may be perceived by others to be disabled and subsequently suffer from employment discrimination even though their condition does not necessarily prevent them from performing major life activities.[7,11]

A highly controversial issue has emerged relative to the third guideline. Obesity as a disability or impairment has spurred intense debate. It potentially ranks as one of the most controversial ADA topics because being overweight is often perceived as being an individual's choice rather than an uncontrollable disability. Although EEOC guidelines in terms of the ADA do not specifically identify obesity as a disability, the condition has been considered a disabling factor in some circumstances.[3] They have, however, determined that individuals who are more than 100% of the normal weight for their specific height may potentially receive protection from discriminatory practices under the ADA. Weight can also be an ADA consideration if it can be linked to a specific medical disorder, which is typically already considered an ADA sanctioned disability.[7]

The 2008 amendments placed a new, significant requirement on employers and the courts in deciding whether an individual can be considered sufficiently disabled to receive protection under the ADA. Employers and courts must now ignore any mitigating measures, such as medications, prosthetics, hearing aids, and such when examining an individual to determine whether a disability exists. This can be of major significance regarding individuals whose continuing ability to function depends largely on medication, since the law now requires courts and employers to consider every disability *in its untreated state.*

The ADA states that impairment or disability alone does not constitute a disability that is under the protection of ADA. The impact of an individual's disability must go beyond the inability to fulfill job duties with or without reasonable accommodation. To be considered a disability that receives protection under ADA, it must impact the individual on a personal level as well. It must prevent the person from effectively performing one or more "major life activities." If normal daily activities are not substantially limited by disability, individuals cannot find refuge from the ADA for disability-related employment actions or label the employer's actions as discriminatory due to disability. In essence, the legal system has determined that if a person can function normally in day-to-day living, that person can function normally at work as well.[1]

The amendments of 2008 have made it easier for individuals to find refuge under the ADA by including a thorough and exhaustive list of major life activities, including caring for oneself, performing manual tasks, eating, sleeping, reading, concentrating, thinking, communicating, and working. The ADA now also expressly states that the operation of any major bodily function is considered a major life activity. At present almost any function or activity one can think of can be identified as a "major life activity."

Impairments may include physiological disorders or conditions, cosmetic disfigurements, anatomical loss affecting one or more of the individual's numerous body systems, or any mental or psychological disorder. The ADA also specifies a number of conditions that are not regarded as disabilities. Those specifically *excluded* from ADA protection include the following:

- Homosexuality and bisexuality (some state and local legislation may protect against discrimination based on sexual orientation)[7]
- Gender-identity disorders, not created by a physical impairment or disorder related to sexual behavior such as transvestitism or transsexualism[7]
- Voyeurism[6]
- Compulsive gambling, pyromania, kleptomania[7]
- Certain disorders resulting from current illegal drug usage such as psychoactive substance abuse[7]
- Drug addicts who have successfully dealt with their addiction and have no further or continuing drug problems are not considered disabled under the ADA[7]

Each of the exclusions listed previously are controversial in terms of their level of protection under ADA. The court system attempts to use the exclusions as a guideline for ADA rulings. For example these guidelines were helpful when a disability discrimination suit was brought up by an employee who tested positive for cocaine during a routine drug test given at work. After testing positive for the drug, the employee was referred by his supervisor to the organization's Employee Assistance Program (EAP) and he was offered time off from work in order to seek treatment.

When the employee returned to work, he alleged that coworkers were accusing him of being a drug user, which he felt was creating a disability-based hostile work environment. He sued under ADA. However, the courts dismissed the case because the individual could not produce any evidence indicating that he had any *current* drug issues. Furthermore, his daily life activities were not impaired by his alleged condition. The courts did not argue that the employee potentially felt hostility at work. However, since he did not have a *current* drug addiction, he could not be considered disabled. Therefore, he was not allowed to claim that the hostility was based on a disability-related issue.[12]

Another defining aspect that aids in determining disability is the duration, or the anticipated duration of the impairment. Injuries such as a broken leg may be problematic and disabling for several weeks but are typically not considered a disability. The ADA indicates that temporary and nonchronic impairments of short duration without long-term or permanent impact are, in fact, not considered disabilities.

The 2008 amendments placed more emphasis on episodic illness and on veterans returning home from the war.[5] Impairments that are "episodic or in remission" may still be considered disabling if, when active, they limit a major life activity. It falls to the employer to determine whether intermittent or episodic impairments could rise to the level of true disability and treat employees accordingly.

Identifying employees who have disabilities is a complex responsibility. Some impairments may not be easily detected and some may be visually apparent. Typically, it is the employee's responsibility to make his or her disability known to the employer and to ask or specify if accommodations are needed.[1] However, employees do not always eagerly report their disabilities to their employers. This has been especially true regarding mental health issues. However, experts feel that the reduction of the stigmas associated with some disabling conditions, such as being bipolar, increases the likelihood that employees will readily disclose their ailments to their employers. Reduced stigmas, the public's expanded knowledge of ADA rights, and the lucrative payouts received when cases are successfully defended are all believed to make reporting disabilities much less intimidating.[13]

Until an employee notifies the employer about a disability, that person is to be treated like all other employees. Managers are not expected and are typically not advised to ask employees about a disability even if one is suspected. This action alone has been associated with discrimination and unfair treatment.[1] However, like most laws, these guidelines are somewhat ambiguous. Although employers are not obligated to ask if a disability exists, healthcare managers should carefully consider how to handle obvious mental health issues. If the mental ailment is obvious, a review of case law indicates that employers cannot use the defense that they "did not know." An employee's failure to notify the employer about a mental health issue will not provide a suitable defense for healthcare managers who are attempting to avoid disability discrimination charges. This is particularly true if an employee poses a direct threat to others.[13]

Essential Functions of the Job

The ADA offers protection for individuals with disabilities who are either employed or potentially employable. It is important to make sure healthcare managers fully understand that the ADA protects disabled individuals who are *qualified* for their positions. A qualified individual is considered as one who can perform the essential functions of the job with or without reasonable accommodation. The person must have the required skills, academic background, and experience to effectively perform the applicable position. A job function is considered essential if and when:

1. That specific function is the reason the position exists,
2. There are a limited number of other employees capable of performing that specific function, and
3. The individual's expertise is the reason for being hired.[6,11]

It is not the intention of the ADA for disabled individuals to be given or allowed to maintain jobs if the disability or impairment prevents performance of the essential functions of the job. Although the ADA protects qualified individuals with disabilities, it does not require an employer to participate in employment transactions with individuals (even disabled individuals) who are not qualified for the position. In other words, being disabled does not immediately and solely qualify an individual for a specific job.[7]

Healthcare managers are not required to lower existing performance standards of the position or to refrain from testing the disabled employee. The key in this instance is that the tests or standards must be uniformly applied to all employees regardless of race, religion, age, gender, religion, and disability. The standards must also be valid indicators that can be appropriately tied to outcomes such as productivity, performance, or patient care.[6]

Individuals who cannot fulfill the essential job duties of the positions are not considered qualified for the jobs and in fact could be considered *disqualified*.[8] For example, when a blind woman applied for a position as a bartender, she was rejected. She sued under ADA. The employer's defense was that she could not carry out the essential job functions of the position because her disability prevented her from effectively recognizing underage or intoxicated patrons. The courts found the employer's defense authentic and ruled against the blind applicant.[14]

In some instances, seniority takes precedence over disability. In other words, disabled workers are not guaranteed to be automatically given those jobs that have been created more specifically for senior members of the workforce.[15] Furthermore, employers are not required to terminate another employee in order to accommodate a disabled individual, and they are not mandated to reduce their qualifications or change what they deem is an essential job function to accommodate a disabled individual.[8, 16]

Physical examinations are often a way that employers determine whether an individual can effectively perform the essential functions of the job. Although, physical examinations cannot be conducted until after a job offer has been extended, employers can typically retract a job offer if the individual is found to be incapable of completing the essential functions of the job.

An individual cannot be refused employment solely because an impairment reduces or prevents adequate performance of a minor, or nonessential, job activity. The individual who cannot complete the essential job functions cannot be considered qualified for the job. Prudent managers may still attempt to determine if the essential functions of the job can be performed with a reasonable accommodation by the disabled person. This is only possible if the essential functions of each position within the organization have been clearly defined.[1]

Employers are expected to be able to produce factual information considering how they determined the essential job functions of the position. The information needs to be precise and accurate in order for essential job functions to be legally defensible.[16] This is essential in today's litigious environment and given the speculations that a significant rise in disability claims and subsequent reasonable accommodation inquiries is on the horizon.[13] Should the need to provide documentation for a manager's decision regarding a disability issue arise, the EEOC will want to know things such as what the essential job functions of the position are, how those functions were determined, and how much time an employee spends on each of the essential job functions.[16]

Determining the essential functions of each position within the organization is imperative in deciding who is qualified and who is not qualified for each position. This provides a positive argument attesting to the need for accurate and up-to-date job descriptions that effectively define the essential functions of every job. Job descriptions act as a defensible mechanism by which claims of disability discrimination can be thwarted since they clearly define the essential job functions and requisite competencies.[6]

In order to develop legally defensible job descriptions, healthcare managers need to fully understand the competencies required and outcomes expected of every position in every department. If an employer can state and demonstrate that the disabled individual was not capable of performing the essential job functions and competencies, then it is likely that allegations of disability discrimination would be unfounded.[16]

However, it cannot be assumed that everything on a particular job description is essential to the job. Managers have a propensity to overuse the essential job function as their only defense, hoping to exclude those that cannot perform every aspect of a job. This strategy can prove costly. For example, an assistant manager for a well-known drug store had a serious automobile accident that resulted in both of her arms being fractured. She returned to work after numerous surgeries, but her left hand and arm were completely nonfunctional and her right arm required the use of a brace. Her activities of daily life were diminished in that she could not shower or dress herself, which substantiated her claim for disability. Doctors released her back to work with a 5-pound lifting restriction but the company refused to allow her return stating that she could never perform the essential functions required of an assistant manager. She sued under ADA. A review of the assistant manager's job description revealed that only 1 out of 23 activities actually required lifting of 5 pounds or more. The courts sided with the disabled employee stating that a reasonable accommodation could be found to fulfill the one activity which required lifting of 5 pounds or more.[16]

Duties of a physical nature are particularly scrutinized by the EEOC in terms of their ADA implications. It is frequently advisable to alter certain job duties to accommodate an individual who can perform all of the essential functions of the job but is hampered in performance of some nonessential function. For example, consider a position in which the incumbent must ordinarily spend 95% of the time generating reports at a computer station and the remaining 5% of the time delivering reports. A rearrangement of duties could place the report delivery, nonessential in the primary task of generating the reports, with another person if the position is to be filled by a qualified individual who is impaired in the activity of walking.

It would be wise for healthcare managers to clearly substantiate the physical demands required by each position such as lifting, standing, bending, and walking. Also of interest to the EEOC will be the types of work surfaces an employee is likely to encounter and any secondary devices used such as ladders. They will want each of these items to correlate with time frames such as occasional, frequent, or constant.[8]

Even if a manager can demonstrate that an employee was not capable of performing the essential functions of the job, it may be necessary to further justify the decision by clearly showing that the actions taken were reasonably necessary and driven by the responsibility to ensure normal business operations. Healthcare managers should be prepared to demonstrate how "factors other than disability" guide their decisions. Using this defense helps to demonstrate that the decisions of the manager were reasonable due to some factor, such as patient safety or poor performance, other than the individual's disability.[6]

Reasonable Accommodation

When an employee is unable to perform the functions of the job as it is currently designed, the healthcare manager must consider making a reasonable accommodation for the disabled worker. Reasonable accommodation simply means changing the work environment or the application process so that a disabled individual could receive an equal employment opportunity. There are three categories of reasonable accommodation that include:

1. Changing a job application process in order to ensure that those with disabilities have equal opportunity to participate in the application process and to be fairly considered for employment. This might include modifications such as larger print on application forms or relocating testing processes to accessible areas.

2. Changing physical components of the job which will enable the disabled employee to perform the essential functions of the position or gain access to the workplace. This might include changes to work hours or larger-button touch-tone telephones.

3. Providing disabled employees with equal access to benefits and privileges of employment.[11] Examples of this may include removing shrubbery that obstructs walkways or replacing small knobs with switches.[11]

The first category of reasonable accommodation dealing with the application process is the source of many ADA allegations. Even applications submitted to medical licensing boards have been heavily scrutinized and shown to include many background and interview questions that are perceivably impermissible in terms of ADA appropriateness. A 2005 study indicates that 96% of all medical licensing board applications reviewed contained questions pertaining to the physical ability, mental health, or substance abuse history of the applicant.[13] This is a risky strategy and most experts will agree that questions or statements about health, disabilities, medical history, or worker's compensation claims should be removed from all application materials.[6]

However, interviewing and selecting employment candidates is a legally charged area in terms of ADA. Employers are strictly prohibited from making preemployment inquiries about an individual's disability or from inquiring about an individual's potential medical conditions. Wal-Mart Corporation was ordered to pay over $6 million in resolution of charges filed under the ADA. The retail icon allegedly had ADA-related statements on a hiring questionnaire that was used in the mid-1990s.[17]

ADA regulations can become considerably complicated for both employer and prospective candidate in this regard. If a prospective employee comes to the interview in a wheelchair, it may be obvious that the person has some type of disability. In such cases, it may prove virtually impossible for the healthcare manager *not* to wonder how the disability will impact the individual's future job performance. However, this would violate ADA regulations.[18]

If it is any consolation to employers, prospective job candidates with disabilities are often uncomfortable with the situation as well. Individuals with disabilities often find that they are in a no-win situation in terms of job interviewing. Some may get through an initial phone interview successfully, but the face-to-face interview is often entirely different. This is especially true of disabilities that are visually evident. An example of this is an individual with multiple sclerosis (MS). Many individuals in an advanced state of MS exhibit visible imbalances in their gait. It can be visually evident that there is a health issue. Prospective employees who try to be completely open with employers about their disabilities often times end up rejected. This happens despite the fact that they are otherwise qualified. However, the manager's concern about issues such as extended absences and escalating healthcare costs illegally cause the employer to find other reasons to excuse the candidate from the candidacy pool.

Like those attempting to be open about their disabilities, the interview process is filled with complexities for those who decide they will exercise their rights under ADA not to discuss their disability. Although ADA guidelines state that disabled individuals do not have to answer illegal questions regarding their disabilities, job candidates feel obligated to answer for fear that their silence will make them appear as if they are hiding something or that they are uncooperative.

Despite ADA protection, many highly qualified individuals with disabilities are illegally rejected for employment because of their impairments. To compound the issues involved with being rejected by employers due to disability, these individuals are often refused financial assistance from Social Security Disability Insurance (SSDI) because they technically are capable of working. A person who is capable of working cannot be considered disabled but may not be able to get a job because of a disability. This is an unfortunate circumstance and perhaps a foundational reason for ADA protection.[18]

Although employers are prohibited from asking disability-related questions, they can ask questions about the individual's ability to perform the essential job functions. For example, employers are generally prohibited from asking if an employee or prospective employee is being treated for any health problems and from inquiring about the existence, nature, or severity of a disability. This would include asking about any previous history of Workers' Compensation claims. However, employers can ask individuals to describe or demonstrate how they would perform job functions.[6]

Determining what reasonable accommodation actually means in terms of an employer's responsibility is still a controversial subject. The basic guideline that has been set forth is that if the cost of the accommodation does not outweigh the benefits associated with having the disabled employee then it is the expectation that a reasonable accommodation will be made.[6] The goal is to make both the facility and the position accessible to the disabled individual.[8]

It is the *employer's* responsibility to provide reasonable accommodations to the disabled employee. For example, if an employee has a hearing impairment it may be suitable in some instances to use a pencil and paper to convey messages. However, other circumstances may require other forms of accommodation such as a sign language interpreter. This type of accommodation would be expected under ADA as long as providing the interpreter did not create an undue burden on the employer's operating costs and the employee was otherwise qualified to perform the duties of the position. Some employers have attempted to pass the costs of accommodations on to the disabled employees by reducing their salary. In the previous scenario, the costs of the interpreter cannot be passed on to the employee in any form.[4]

Employers are required to provide a reasonable accommodation to individuals who are otherwise qualified for the job unless doing so presents an undue hardship on the organization.[6] This option is only mandated when the employee meets the previously discussed criteria associated with a disabling impairment. However, in terms of reasonable accommodation, only the first two criteria typically apply:

1. The individual must have a physical or mental impairment that limits one or more of the major life activities, or

2. There must be a record of said impairment.

The ADA may offer disability classification for those fitting the third criterion identified as:

3. Regarded as having an impairment.

However, the disfigured burn victim mentioned earlier will enjoy little mandated protection in terms of reasonable accommodation from the ADA. Protection for such individuals may more likely be found within the Rehabilitation Act of 1973.[11]

Undue Hardship or Undue Burden

The ADA provides the undue hardship defense as a means by which employers can excuse themselves from ADA sanctions when they elect to forgo reasonable accommodations for a disabled employee or job candidate.[8] This aspect of ADA regulation is complicated since a precise and workable definition of undue hardship is not provided by the ADA as a form of guidance for employers. Further complicating the issue is that the EEOC bases its decisions on a case-by-case basis, which varies widely. Undue hardship, also known as undue burden, is one that:

- Creates a significant expense,
- Is excessively difficult,
- Causes an extensive disruption, and
- Creates a fundamental change to the nature and operations of business. [3,19]

The standard for claiming an undue hardship is high and healthcare managers should not make this claim lightly. Studies indicate that the average costs for employers to accommodate the disabled are as follows:

- 31% experienced no cost
- 19% experienced costs of $1.00 to $50.00
- 19% experienced costs of $51.00 to $500.00
- 19% experienced costs of $501.00 to $1000.00
- 11% experienced costs of $1001.00 to $5000.00
- 1% experienced costs of $5000.00 or more[20]

Given this information, it would appear that a high percentage of reasonable accommodations are relatively feasible for most organizations in terms of associated costs. Therefore, it is easy to understand that undue hardship claims may be closely scrutinized and evaluated by the EEOC for authenticity. Furthermore, EEOC bases its rulings on *all* resources and assets available to the facility in question. Just because making a reasonable accommodation is cost prohibitive for the department does not mean that it creates an undue hardship for the whole facility.[21] The EEOC will also determine whether the facility making the undue burden claim is part of a larger corporation that perhaps would not be unduly burdened by making necessary accommodations for a disabled worker.[19]

Obviously, caution should be exercised when stating that reasonable accommodations will cause an excessive financial burden. Employers using the undue hardship defense are still required under the ADA to seek alternative options, which, to the maximum extent possible, ensure both effective business operations and appropriate consideration for the disabled individual.[21] For example, reasonable accommodation could include redesigning the position, restructuring job assignments, modifying work schedules, or modifying or acquiring equipment or other devices to assist the individual in effectively performing the duties of the job.[6, 8] This may involve modifications that are relatively easy and not cost prohibitive. Some examples might include resolutions as simple as installing entry and exit ramps, repositioning work stations, widening doorways, or installing grab bars in restroom stalls.[8] Other reasonable accommodations might include modified examinations, disability-specific training materials, or revised organizational policies.

Nonessential duties of the job that might exclude disabled individuals should be carefully considered and removed from that job if possible. Obviously, the job duties that are removed must be covered by someone else within the organization. This is an acceptable resolution to a reasonable accommodation if moving the job duties to another employee does not present an undue hardship to the employer. For example, a coding specialist not physically capable of lifting 10 pound boxes of medical charts may still be a highly qualified and skilled medical coder. ADA notwithstanding, it would be unfortunate to lose a talented coder simply because that person cannot lift a box because of a disability. It is hoped that good management sense would seek a solution to retaining this employee even if there were not a federal mandate such as ADA.

In circumstances such as the foregoing, managers would be urged to consider job description trade-offs that may remove the nonessential job duty of lifting boxes from the disabled individual and place that responsibility with another employee. Job responsibilities should be equally dispersed between disabled employees and non-disabled employees by restructuring job duties based around the essential functions of the position and the capabilities and skill levels of all employees. This is not to say that lifting boxes may not be an essential job duty for some positions. Obviously, lifting boxes may very well be an essential job duty for someone on the loading dock responsible for unloading trucks that are delivering materials and supplies.

Excluding the responsibility of lifting boxes from a position for which it is an essential job duty is not required by ADA. An example that demonstrates this especially well involves an employee with a back condition who worked as a door greeter for a retail store. Because of her back condition she asked if she could sit on a stool while working. The store rejected her request and she sued under ADA. The company's decision was upheld by the federal district court. It was determined that part of the essential job duties of being a door greeter included acting in an aggressively hospitable manner, which could not be done while sitting on a stool. The courts supported the employer's claims that standing was an essential job function and made their ruling accordingly.[22]

Readily Achievable

Along with the category of reasonable accommodation is the issue of accommodations related to building structure, layout, furnishings, equipment, and accessibility. It most cases it is prudent for employers to make their facilities as ADA compliant and accessible as possible by carefully considering all aspects of their facility. However, the ADA does not require a facility to be totally rebuilt to accommodate employees with disabilities. For example, a facility located at the top of a hill without an easily accessible path of travel from the employee parking lot does not need to tear down the building and rebuild it at the bottom of the hill. If it is easy to accomplish, without too much of a financial obligation to the employer, it would be prudent to make more accessible parking closer to the facility. This would only be a feasible resolution if constructing a new parking lot was readily achievable based on a variety of factors including, but not limited to, the facility itself, the land, building codes and regulations, and the financial obligation to the employer.

There may be other accommodations that are more readily achievable, such as an employee shuttle charged with the responsibility of transporting employees up a hill. A solution such as this might be a more financially prudent and practical consideration. Again, this is only required by ADA if it does not pose a significant or undue hardship on the employer. It is always sensible to explore any and every potential reasonable accommodation or readily achievable solution. Employers should consult a tax attorney or the Internal Revenue Service regarding business deductions that may be available for those trying to make their facilities more ADA friendly.[21]

Direct Threat

Another controversial issue recognized by the ADA is direct threat. This may be particularly important in the healthcare field given the nature of the work and the fact that unqualified or incapable individuals in patient care areas could be detrimental to the well-being of those they serve. A direct threat is stated to exist when a considerable risk of significant harm to the health or safety of an individual or others that cannot be effectively alleviated with a reasonable accommodation. For example, a manager would not be forced by the ADA to hire a surgical nurse disabled with narcolepsy who commonly and unpredictably becomes unconscious. Being alert at all times during surgical procedures would be considered an essential function of the job. Furthermore, finding a reasonable accommodation for this individual may prove impossible. It may be simply too impractical to have a surgical nurse disabled by a condition such as narcolepsy.[3]

Direct threat must be based on an individual assessment of each employee. If the manager determines that an employee's disability poses a direct threat to others, a specific behavior felt to pose that threat must be clearly identified. Merely having a disability, especially if the disability is related to mental health, does not automatically mean that a direct threat exists. Furthermore, case law indicates that employees taking prescribed medication for their disabilities cannot be automatically assumed by their employers to pose a direct threat. This is true even if the employee operates machinery. Employers often want to claim that taking the medication reduces the concentration or coordination levels of the employee. These types of defenses have been unsuccessfully used by employers.

Although employers cannot assume that someone taking medication poses a threat to others, they typically are not expected to be responsible for making sure employees take their prescribed medicine. This does not fall under a reasonable accommodation that is typically required of employers by the ADA. However, modifying work schedules, providing a career coach, changing management styles, or reducing noise and distractions may be reasonable accommodations which managers might need to consider.[13]

Direct threat provisions within the ADA include no mandate to place disabled individuals in positions where their impairment may present potential harm to others. For example, an employee threatened to throw one of her fellow workers out of a window. After completing a 10-day suspension the employee was diagnosed as paranoid. Upon her return to work, she threatened her supervisor and promised to kill her. When she was fired, she sued under the ADA. Her case was dismissed because the courts determined that although she did have a debilitating mental illness, the ADA does not typically protect employees who threaten other employees.[23]

Another example of direct threat in the courts involved an employee who alleged that his supervisor violated the ADA by forcing him to take a fitness-for-duty exam. The supervisor requested the employee be tested after the employee made statements that he would "go postal" if he had problems at work. The supervisor, concerned that the employee might pose a threat to others, put the employee on paid leave insisting that the employee take a mental fitness-for-duty test to determine any potential threats. The employee took the test but refused to disclose the results to the employer. Therefore, for the safety of other employees, the supervisor felt obligated to terminate the disturbed employee. The employee sued under ADA, but the supervisor claimed that the exam was a business necessity and was needed in order to determine if the subordinate posed a threat to himself or others. The court sided with the employer, stating that the mental evaluation was a true business necessity and that the company had an obligation to investigate all threats in order to assure the safety of all employees.[24]

The ADA does not specifically address the issue of direct threat when the potential for harm may be toward the disabled individuals themselves. However, employers are not mandated by ADA to allow a disabled employee to demand a position that poses a significant life-threatening consequence to others or to the disabled individual.[25]

ADA and Mental Impairments

The National Institute of Mental Health (NIMH) indicates that one in every five adults in the United States is plagued with a mental disorder every year. Depression, bipolar disorder, obsessive-compulsive disorder, and schizophrenia are among the 10 top leading causes of disability in the United States. The following provides an overview of the number of mental health discrimination claims reported from 1992 through 1999:

- 7820 claims associated with depression
- 2748 claims associated with anxiety
- 2050 claims associated with bipolar disorder
- 440 claims associated with schizophrenia[13]

An individual is considered to have a disability if the person has an impairment (physical or mental) that substantially reduces their life activities. The number of disability claims associated with mental impairments has been steadily increasing over the years.[6] Between 1993 and 1997, 13% of all ADA complaints filed were related to emotional or mental disorders.[7]

Numbers such as these are expected to increase as the population as a whole ages because there is a perceivable correlation between age and mental health. Some mental health illnesses have become excessively common, such as depression, which is eloquently referred to as "the common cold" of mental health illnesses. This demonstrates the gravity of the mental health problem in America because many individuals with mental health impairments will be applying for employment or are currently employed. Managers may be unaware of how many current and potential employees already qualify for protection under the ADA due to mental health-related reasons.[13]

The complexities of mental health-related issues are obvious. However, the ambiguous environment is one that healthcare managers will find themselves mandated to navigate. This is largely due to the increased number of allegations associated with disability discrimination.

The number of ADA-related complaints moving through the court system is overwhelming. Traditionally, ADA plaintiffs have had a difficult time prevailing and the decisions of employers have been largely supported by the courts. Employees have not been able to sufficiently demonstrate that they are truly disabled or that they are truly qualified to do the job.

However, when employees win disability discrimination lawsuits, they typically receive large settlements and the ramifications for employers who violate the rights of employee with mental health impairments are particularly intense.[6,13] The monetary awards given to those who successfully present an ADA allegation can be financially severe. In 1999, approximate financial awards given for alleged ADA violations against employers for violating mental health disabilities were as follows:

- Depression: $3,494,922.00 was awarded in 185 individual cases; an average of $18,891.00 per case.
- Anxiety: $2,004,889.00 was awarded in 65 individual cases; an average of $30,844.00 per case.
- Bipolar: $777,914.00 was awarded in 57 individual cases; an average of $13,647.00 per case.
- Schizophrenia: $71,566.00 awarded in 10 individual cases; an average of $7156.00 per case.[16]

Because of the complexity of ADA regulations, in 1997, the EEOC issued new guidelines specific to mental health regulations.[13] In addition to those afflictions previously mentioned, a mental impairment under the ADA includes any mental or psychological disorder. These impairments may include conditions such as major depression, anxiety or panic disorders, and obsessive-compulsive disorders. Employers are urged to consider that normally undesirable issues such as chronic lateness, hostility toward fellow workers, and poor judgment may be linked to mental impairments that may be protected under the ADA.[6]

Avoiding ADA Allegations

Of foremost importance in the effort to prevent ADA allegations or charges is the creation of a work environment that is tolerant of individual differences. Sensitivity training and the creation of awareness in the general employee population are steps in the right direction. Managers should understand and account for the feelings other employees may have regarding the reasonable accommodations provided for disabled individuals. These accommodations may be resented by others as special privileges. This resentment can subsequently create a work environment that makes the disabled employee feel unwanted or even threatened. Attempts should be made by the manager to focus other employees on the disabled individual's skills and talents as opposed to the person's impairment. This needs to be done without making the disabled individual feel singled out or treated differently. As can be imagined, this requires delicate balance and managerial finesse.[13]

Conclusion

Both employees and employers face many complex challenges in terms of ADA legislation. Preventing allegations of discriminatory activities that fall under the protective umbrella of ADA is challenging. As previously noted, the ADA is somewhat elusive with a case-by-case philosophy in terms of employer application. However, managers should make every effort possible to comply with ADA mandates and the expectations outlined in this civil rights statute.

It is vital for healthcare managers to fully explore the issues faced by their organizations in terms of disability discrimination protection and to properly interpret and implement appropriate EEOC guidelines. As the workplace becomes increasingly complex and diversified, healthcare managers must move cautiously into the ambiguous areas associated with disabled workers. Individuals within the organization charged with the responsibility of assisting in the personnel process must be fully educated about the legislation that pertains to all forms of discrimination. Managers may need to identify and modify all of the functions associated with employee transactions to avoid discriminatory actions. They must be fully aware of illegal interview questions, unlawful testing processes, and other discriminatory practices. Furthermore, managers should routinely conduct a full assessment of personnel policies including hiring, application processes, selection, testing, promotion, compensation, disciplinary actions, and termination. Understanding such concepts as reasonable accommodation and essential job functions is a positive beginning. This will require an extensive review of job descriptions and the identification of essential job functions and nonessential job functions. Unfortunately, this review is not a static event to occur only once. Revisiting personnel policies and procedures is a dynamic process that perpetually needs ongoing managerial attention.[6] Special attention should be placed on following ADA regulations pertaining to mental health illnesses which are expected to increase rapidly over the next few decades. This is especially true given the expanded knowledge base regarding ADA rights that current employees seemingly possess.[13]

Questions for Review and Discussion

1. How can some of the activities that are legitimately part of a particular job and are included in the job description not be considered essential functions of the job?

2. Cite one particular type of impairment and describe how a person so impaired may be hired for one kind of job but legitimately rejected for another kind of job.

3. Why was the Americans with Disabilities Act (ADA) considered necessary when disabled persons were already protected under Title VII of the Civil Rights Act of 1964?

4. What is most likely the only interview question that can be asked relative to an applicant's physical condition?

5. When may an individual exhibiting some obvious impairment not be able to call upon the protection of the ADA?

6. Provide a specific example of an "impairment" that is excluded from ADA protection and explain why this is so.

7. Why is there not an all-inclusive list of disabilities eligible for protection under the ADA?

8. Provide an example of the circumstances under which a particular requested accommodation may not be considered reasonable.

9. Explain why an individual whose impairment prohibits employment in a certain capacity may nevertheless be ineligible for other considerations such as Social Security Disability.

10. How does the ADA specify that an apparent direct threat should be assessed?

References

1. Fallon, L., & McConnell, C. (2007). *Human resource management in health care: Principles and practice.* Sudbury, MA: Jones and Bartlett.
2. Fisher, R. (1995). *Evaluating social policy.* Chicago: Nelson-Hall Publishers.
3. Jones, N. (2003). *The Americans with Disabilities Act (ADA): Overview, regulations, and interpretations.* New York: Novinka Books.
4. United States Department of Justice. (2002). *Commonly asked questions about the Americans with Disabilities Act and law enforcement.* Washington, DC: Civil Rights Division, Disability Rights Section.
5. HR Specialist. (2009). *Good news: ADA amendments can't be invoked retroactively.* Available at: http://www.thehrspecialist.com/article.aspx?articleid=28699. Accessed October 15, 2009.
6. Dressler, G. (2003). *Human resource management* (9th ed.). Upper Saddle River, NJ: Prentice Hall.
7. Fried, B., & Fottler, M. (2008). *Human resources in healthcare: Managing for success* (3rd ed.). Arlington, VA: Health Administration Press.
8. McConnell, C. (2006). *Umiker's management skills for the new health care supervisor* (4th ed.). Sudbury, MA: Jones and Bartlett.
9. O'Brien, R. (2001). *Crippled justice: The history of modern disability policy in the workplace.* Chicago: University of Chicago Press.
10. Mueller, P. (2007). *Access for all: A policy analysis of the Americans with Disability Act.* (Unpublished master's thesis). University of Northern Colorado, Greeley, CO.
11. United States Department of Agriculture. (n.d.). *Reasonable accommodation procedures.* Available at: http://www.da.usda.gov/oo/target/subjects/at/addlcap/foreword.htm. Accessed January 6, 2010.
12. HR Specialist. (2009). *Recovered addict not automatically disabled.* Available at: http://www.thehrspecialist.com/article.aspx?articleid=28748. Accessed November 16, 2009.
13. Schroeder, R., Brazeau, C., Zackin, F., Rovi, S., Dickey, J., Johnson, M., et al. (2009). Do state medical board applications violate the Americans with Disabilities Act? *Academic Medicine, 85*(6), 776–781.

14. Semler, R. (1998). Developing management incentives that drive results. *Compensation and Benefits Review, 30*(4), 41–48.

15. Associated Press. (2002, April 30). Seniority outweighs disability, Court Says. *Democrat & Chronicle.*

16. HR Specialist. (2009). *Don't nickel and dime ADA accommodations: Everything can't be essential to the job.* Available at: http://www.thehrspecialist.com/article.aspx?articleid=28759. Accessed November 16, 2009.

17. Wright, T. (2002). ADA restricts medical inquiries. *Credit Union Magazine, 68*(4), 89.

18. Shaw, K. (2008). The disability rights movement: The ADA today. *Momentum, 1*(4), 20–25.

19. United Nations General Assembly. (2006, January–February). *Concept of reasonable accommodation.* Seventh Session of the Ad Hoc Committee on a Comprehensive and Integral International Convention on the Protection and Promotion of the Rights and Dignity of Persons with Disabilities. New York. Available at: www.un.org/esa/socdev/enable/rights/ahc7bkgrndra.htm. Accessed January 6, 2010.

20. Goldstein, M., Simonds, C., & Sanders, C. (1995). *Succeeding together: People with disabilities in the workplace.* Available at: www.csun.edu/~sp20558/dis/reasonable.html. Accessed January 6, 2010.

21. United States and National Rehabilitation Hospital. (1994). *Answers to questions commonly asked by hospitals and health care providers: ADA, the Americans with Disabilities Act (ADA).* Washington, DC: National Rehabilitation Hospital, ADA Compliance Program.

22. Borofsky, G., Bielema, M., & Hoffman, J. (1993). Accidents, turnover, and use of a pre-employment screening interview. *Psychological Reports, 73*, 1067–1076.

23. Reese, G., & Waltemath, J. (1996). *Workers' compensation manual for managers and supervisors* (2nd ed.). Chicago: CCH Incorporated.

24. Institute of Business Publications. (2009). Worker says he'll 'go postal,' then sues when supervisor orders mental-fitness test. *Legal Alert for Supervisors, 5*(103), 1–2.

25. Associated Press. (2002, June 11). Top court disallows dangerous jobs for disabled. *Democrat & Chronicle.*

Chapter 5

The Civil Rights Act of 1964: Changing the Face of Employment

Eric Matthews, PhD, *Assistant Professor, College of Applied Sciences and Arts, Southern Illinois University Carbondale, Carbondale, Illinois*

Chapter Objectives

- Review the history of proposed and unsuccessful legislation that preceded passage of the Civil Rights Act of 1964, the country's first significant legislation addressing discrimination in all aspects of employment.
- Provide an understanding of Title VII of the Civil Rights Act as it affects managers and their role in employment processes.
- Review subsequent legislation that effectively augmented and strengthened the Civil Rights Act, including the Age Discrimination in Employment Act (ADEA) of 1967, the Equal Employment Opportunity Act of 1972, the Civil Rights Act of 1991, and others.
- Provide guidelines intended to assist employers and their managers and recruiters in avoiding acts of unintentional discrimination.
- Introduce the Equal Employment Opportunity Commission (EEOC) as the enforcement agency for the Civil Rights Act of 1964 and related legislation.

Introduction

Just before 10:00 in the morning on June 10, 1964, Senator Robert Byrd finished an address to the US Senate that had rambled on longer than 14 hours. He was the last in a long line of senators who had stood to oppose the impending Civil Rights Act that was presently before the Senate for debate. Armed with the votes necessary to end a filibuster that was taking place on the bill, Hubert Humphrey, the bill's manager, called for cloture (the means of overcoming a filibuster) on the bill. Seldom had such a measure succeeded, and never had a call for cloture succeeded relevant to a bill on civil rights; however, for the first time in 37 years, the cloture measure passed and brought to an end the debate on the Civil Rights Act. Previously, filibusters had been the primary way southern Democrats had blocked attempted legislation on civil rights. With the cloture measure passed, the present filibuster, which had lasted 57 days, was brought to an end. Nine days later, the Senate voted on and passed the Civil Rights Act, bringing to fruition the implied intent of the Fourteenth Amendment to the US Constitution, the equality of all Americans.

History

Public Bill 82-352 was properly called:

> An Act to enforce the constitutional right to vote, to confer jurisdiction upon the district courts of the United States of America to provide relief against discrimination in public accommodations, to authorize the Attorney General to institute suits to protect constitutional rights in public facilities and public education, to extend the Commission on Civil Rights, to prevent discrimination in federally assisted programs, to establish a Commission on Equal Employment Opportunity, and for other purposes.

The bill was formally shortened to, and is still referred to as the Civil Rights Act of 1964. This was not the first attempt by the government of the United States to pass legislation guaranteeing the individual civil rights of American citizens; there had been numerous earlier attempts, all of which had either failed or were ineffective. However, nominal knowledge of these bills is important for a full appreciation of the impact of the 1964 Civil Rights Act.

The first attempt by the Congress to guarantee the civil rights of Americans was passed in 1866, immediately following the Civil War. The 1866 Civil Rights Act (the first act to bear the name "Civil Rights Act") was the initial attempt by Congress to guarantee the rights of freedmen (former slaves) during reconstruction. The act was a direct counter to the Black Codes, which had been enacted by former slave-holding states in the southern United States as a result of the passage of the Thirteenth Amendment to the US Constitution, which forbade slavery. The Black Codes were laws passed at state and local levels in the South to inhibit the ability of former slaves to act as social equals of the whites in those areas; the codes were responsible for suppressing the ability of former slaves to gain equality with whites in the South. With the Civil Rights Bill of 1866, Congress attempted to guarantee the Civil and Legal Equality of most individuals in the United States. It stated that

> All persons born in the United States not subject to any foreign power, excluding Indians not taxed, are hereby declared to be citizens of the United States; and such citizens, of every race and color, without regard to previous condition of slavery or involuntary servitude, except as punishment for crime whereof the party shall have been duly convicted, shall have the same right, in every State and Territory in the United States . . . as is enjoyed by white citizens . . .

When President Andrew Johnson vetoed the bill, Congress overrode it, and on April 9, 1866, the bill became law. While the Civil Rights Act of 1866 was impotent due to lack of enforcement in the targeted South and the inability of those being discriminated against to access legal aid, it was pivotal in that it contained the first major antidiscrimination employment statute when it gave minorities the same rights to "make and enforce contracts," which included employment contracts.

Following the Civil Rights Act of 1866, there was moderate concern (not surprisingly among the southern congressional delegations and the inhabitants of those states) that the government of the United States did not possess the authority to pass laws interpreting the constitutional rights of citizens; however, that was put to rest on July 9, 1868, with the adoption of the Fourteenth Amendment to the Constitution. The Fourteenth Amendment to the Constitution of the United States was, along with the Thirteenth and Fifteenth amendments, one of the reconstruction amendments passed by Congress following the end of the Civil War. Effectively, the Fourteenth Amendment overturned the previous findings of the 1857 US Supreme Court in the case of *Dred Scott v. Sandford*. The primary finding of the Dred Scott case was that people of African descent imported into the United States, along with their descendants, were not extended the rights of citizenship in the United States. The intent of the Fourteenth Amendment was to extend full citizenship to the individuals formerly held as slaves, which would uphold the Civil Rights Act of 1866. Unfortunately, the intent of the amendment and the interpretation of the amendment were entirely different, particularly in the deep South, where racial segregation continued to exist and flourish.

While the intent of the 1866 bill was to aid reconstruction blacks by extending to them citizenship, in reality, it did little toward guaranteeing their civil rights. The Civil Rights Act of 1871 was an attempt to augment this earlier legislation by aiding in the protection of southern blacks from the Ku Klux Klan. However, in the interim, it was broadly interpreted by the various courts of the Federal

Judicial system, and, as such, is important for modern public sector employers. In part, the 1871 act reads that any person who deprives another individual of any rights secured either by the Constitution or the various laws of the land "shall be liable to the party injured in an action at law, suit in equity, or other proper proceeding for redress." As a result, the law is often used to secure the rights of an individual in employment discrimination cases whereby a government entity does not ensure the rights of an individual in determining employment eligibility.

The Civil Rights Act of 1875 is commonly described as the "Separate but Equal" act. It was declared unconstitutional by the US Supreme Court in 1883, but many of the provisions it contained would find their way into the civil rights acts of the 1960s. Perhaps the most important aspect of the Civil Rights Act of 1875 was the guarantee that anyone "within the jurisdiction of the United States shall be entitled to the full and equal enjoyment of the accommodations, advantages, facilities, and privileges of inns, public conveyances on land or water, theaters, and other places of public amusement." The act attempted to guarantee there would be no discrimination against individuals of varying race relative to their activities in daily life. However, the act attempted to regulate the treatment of one individual by another, and, in 1883, it was deemed unconstitutional when the Supreme Court determined that the government did not have the power to regulate the conduct of individuals, and struck down the act.

Following the end of reconstruction in 1877 and the flurry of civil rights legislation that was pursued during the period, it would be more than 80 years before another piece of legislation dealing with civil rights would pass through the Congress. The Civil Rights Act of 1957 was proposed primarily to ensure the voting rights of African Americans by Republican President Dwight Eisenhower. The act was extremely controversial at the time, even among members of the Democratic party. It was sent to committee and amended, altered, and changed until it bore almost no resemblance to its originally intended purpose. However, it made it out of committee and onto the Senate floor for debate. Ultimately, the bill passed, but not before it underwent the longest one-person filibuster in history, which was undertaken by Senator James Strom Thurmond, who rambled on for 24 hours and 18 minutes, reading everything from the Declaration of Independence to random phone books and his grandmother's biscuit recipe. Like most of the preceding civil rights legislation, it was ineffective in scope and implementation. However, there were a number of tenets of the bill that were pivotal in the success of later legislation. The Civil Rights Act of 1957 instituted both the Commission on Civil Rights and the Office of the Assistant Attorney General on Civil Rights. As a result of the formation of these federal departments and offices, the attorney general (William Rogers) created the Civil Rights Division within the Justice Department. This would prove pivotal in defending and upholding the forthcoming legislation on civil rights.

Background for the 1964 Civil Rights Act

It has been noted by many that the Civil Rights Act of 1964 was a landmark in the civil rights movement and the journey toward desegregation and equality that had been in motion since before the Civil War. As has been demonstrated, the 1964 act was the latest in a long line of civil rights legislation. However, the bill was introduced to an America that had changed and was ripe for the philosophies entailed in the act. The bill itself was the culmination of work that had began with the Civil Rights Act of 1866, and was a direct evolution of the Civil Rights Acts of 1957 (the first major bill pertaining to civil rights that had been passed since Reconstruction) and 1960 (also an ineffective bill).

Recognizing the need for racial desegregation and an end to racial oppression, President John F. Kennedy delivered a special message to Congress on February 28, 1963. The message Kennedy delivered called upon Congress to enact civil rights legislation. Kennedy, however, met many obstructions from Congress to this agenda.

A primary obstruction to Kennedy's civil rights initiative was the membership of Congress. In 1963, the Chairman of the House Rules Committee was Howard Smith. Smith was a conservative southern Democrat from Virginia who opposed civil rights legislation with a fervor seldom matched. Any legislation coming out of the House would have to go through the Rules Committee chaired by Smith. Kennedy knew he would have to circumvent Smith, or at least maneuver him into supporting any civil rights legislation.

Concurrently, in the Senate, the Judiciary Committee was headed by another southern Democrat from Mississippi, James Eastland. During his tenure as the Chairman of the Judiciary Committee, Eastland had killed more than 100 proposed civil rights bills. However, the biggest obstacle to a civil rights bill in the Senate was not the Judiciary Committee; rather, it was the ability of the southern Democrats to stage a filibuster. It was their filibustering ability that had dramatically altered the Civil Rights Acts of 1957 and 1960 to the point that they became ineffective. Again, the supporters of the bills altered them to a point they would be acceptable to the southern Democrats so they would allow them to come to a vote. Once the dilution happened, the bills lost their ability to influence the racial situation in the South.

Kennedy also faced a harsh political reality within his own party. He did not have the political capital to expend forcing the bill through without alienating the southern Democratic congressmen. He could not run the risk of separating himself from his party and hope to get any of his other legislation passed, including several arms treaties, which took precedence. As a result of these tribulations, Kennedy was effectively hamstrung and incapable of getting the legislation that he sought through Congress. Therefore, Kennedy was forced to accept implicit defeat. While the bill slogged its way through the outlined congressional quagmire, he simply worked within the bounds of the executive branch by appointing blacks to as many positions as possible within the government and ordering the Justice Department to act on behalf of individuals involved in racial segregation protests.

The bill Kennedy had introduced made its way through the House Judiciary Committee where it received support, primarily from northern and western Democrats. As the bill was reported out of the Judiciary Committee in late November 1963, it was sent to the House Rules Committee where Howard Smith vowed to keep it bottled up (forever if necessary). Thus, Congress was preparing itself for what promised to be an epic fight when Kennedy headed to Texas to begin his reelection campaign.

Obviously, Kennedy never returned from that trip, having been assassinated in Dallas on November 22, 1963. Generally, it was felt that Kennedy's demise spelled doom for the Civil Rights bill, particularly since Lyndon Johnson was a Southern Democrat who was nominally against the civil rights issue. However, what civil rights activists failed to account for was Johnson's desire to win reelection in 1964. Johnson had little time to convince the powerful northern contingent of the Democratic party that a southerner could be an effective party leader. In the Civil Rights Act, he found the perfect catalyst to ingratiate himself with the northern and western liberals that held sway over the Democratic party.

Less than a week after Kennedy's assassination, Johnson told a joint session of Congress "we have talked long enough in this country about equal rights . . . It is time now to write the next chapter and to write it in the books of law." Playing on the sympathies and passions of the assembled Congress, Johnson asked that the civil rights bill be adopted in memory of its slain champion, President Kennedy. Unlike Kennedy, who was constrained trying not to offend members of his party, Johnson threw the presidential weight of the White House behind his bid to successfully pass the Civil Rights Act. Further, he determined that (unlike previous civil rights bills) this bill would transit the Congress without being diluted to appease southern Democrats. Johnson succeeded in all regards and on the same evening, the House of Representatives agreed to the Senate version of the bill, and on July 2, 1964, President Johnson signed into law the Civil Rights Act in a nationally televised event. During the course of his television address, Johnson noted that "Americans of every race and color" had died in defense of the freedoms of the United States. He further noted that Americans believed that all men were created equal, yet they denied men equal treatment and that it was time for that to end. That it was imperative that Americans who were "equal before God shall now also be equal in the polling booths, in the classrooms, in the factories . . ." And with that and a few other remarks, the Civil Rights Act of 1964 passed into law.

The Bill in Action

The Civil Rights Act of 1964 was divided into 10 sections or titles. While Title VII is of the highest consequence in employment law and management, it is important to understand the various other facets of the bill.

Title I pertains to the rights of voters. In effect, the title bars unequal application of voter registration requirements. While Title I did not remove the various ways in which voters could be discriminated against, it stated that so long as all voters were given the same opportunity to vote, it was sufficient in the eyes of the government. In effect, this failed to challenge the notion of voter qualification. By doing that, the bill implied that voting was not an automatic right of citizenship, but that there may be some qualifying factor beyond that base standard. If the qualifying factor (such as a literacy test) were applied equally to all races, that would satisfy the intent of the bill.

Title II of the act provided for "Injunctive Relief Against Discrimination in Places of Public Accommodation." The second section of the act noted that everyone was entitled to equally enjoy the goods and services of public accommodations. This outlawed discrimination in such places as hotels, motels, restaurants, theaters, among others. In actuality, it included any "public accommodation" involved in interstate commerce. Title II notably exempted private clubs, but did not define "private."

Title III enforced desegregation of public facilities. This mandated that both state and municipal governments could not deny access to public facilities on grounds of race, religion, gender, or ethnicity.

Title IV of the bill may have intended to desegregate the public schools of the United States. In reality, the section stated that schools should perform equally within 2 years of the passage of the bill. It allowed the attorney general to file suit against school districts to accomplish this equality.

Title V of the act greatly expanded the Civil Rights Commission that had been inaugurated by the Civil Rights Act of 1957. The section granted additional powers, rules, and procedures to the commission. It also mandated reports to both the president and Congress.

Title VI outlawed discrimination in federally assisted programs. This title clearly stated that anyone, regardless of race, color, or national origin could not be discriminated against by being excluded from programs that received *any* portion of their funding from the federal government. It also said they could not be discriminated against by denying them the benefits of programs that received federal funding.

Title VIII of the act dealt specifically with voter registration and voter statistics. It mandated a compilation of voter registration and voter data in areas that were identified by the Civil Rights Commission. However, it only required such records for elections that had been held since January 1, 1960.

Title IX embraced the lack of a fair trial that certain civil rights plaintiffs were receiving in the South as a result of segregationist judges and all-white juries. It made it substantially easier for civil rights cases to move from state courts where the proceedings would be biased to federal courts. This made it easier for civil rights activists to receive a fair trial in cases involving their actions in pursuit of racial equality.

Title X of the act established the Community Relations Service, a division of the US Department of Justice. Its primary role is to act as a mediator in cases of discrimination arising from breaches of the Civil Rights Act. It also acts to assist state and local governments in preventing or resolving racial and ethnic tensions, incidents and disorders, in addition to restoring racial stability and harmony. See Exhibit 5-1 for a brief outline of the Civil Rights Act of 1964.

Exhibit 5-1

General Outline of the Civil Rights Act of 1964

- Title I barred unequal application of voter registration requirements.
- Title II outlawed discrimination in public accommodations engaged in interstate commerce, except private clubs (e.g., hotels, motels, restaurants, theaters).
- Title III prohibited state and municipal governments from denying access to public facilities on the grounds of race, religion, gender, or ethnicity.
- Title IV encouraged desegregation of public schools.
- Title V expanded the Civil Rights Commission, granting additional power, along with more defined rules and procedures.
- Title VI prevents discrimination by government agencies that receive federal funding.
- Title VII primarily prohibits discrimination by covered employers on the basis of race, color, religion, sex, or national origin.
- Title VIII required compilation of voter registration and voter data in geographic areas that were specified by the Commission on Civil Rights.
- Title IX made it easier for a claimant to move civil rights cases from state courts to federal courts, allowing them to circumvent discriminatory judges and juries.
- Title X established the Community Relations Service, tasked with assisting in community disputes involving claims of discrimination.

Title VII

To define the mandates of Title VII, as has been demonstrated, it is important to understand them in both the context of the time in which they were enacted and as a larger portion of the laws of the United States. According to the US Department of Justice (Civil Rights Division), Title VII of the Civil Rights Act of 1964 (as amended, 42 U.S.C. §2000e, et seq.) prohibits discrimination in employment on the basis of race, sex, national origin, and religion. It also makes it unlawful for any employer to take actions of a retaliatory nature against any person for opposing employment practices that had been made illegal or unlawful by Title VII (i.e., individuals protesting discriminatory hiring and employment practices). Further, Title VII makes it illegal for employers to retaliate against employees for filing a discrimination charge, or for testifying, assisting, or participating in an investigation, proceeding, or hearing being held under the auspices of the enforcement clauses of Title VII.

The exact wording of the bill indicates that it is unlawful for an employer to "fail or refuse to hire or to discharge any individual, or otherwise to discriminate against any individual with respect to his compensation, terms, conditions or privileges or employment, because of such individual's race, color, religion, sex, or national origin." The bill also states that it is against the law for an employer to

> limit, segregate, or classify his employees or applicants for employment in any way which would deprive or tend to deprive any individual of employment opportunities or otherwise adversely affect his status as an employee, because of such individual's race, color, religion, sex, or national origin.

It is important to note that while Title VII is very stringent about what an employer can and cannot do relative to hiring and employing individuals, Title VII only applies to employers having 15 or more employees for every workday in 20 contiguous calendar weeks. These calendar weeks may span multiple calendar years, but they must be consecutive. Simply put, Title VII prohibits workplace harassment and discrimination in businesses with more than 15 employees, educational entities, or any governmental (local, state, or federal) agency. See Exhibit 5-2 for employers who fall under the auspices of the Civil Rights Act of 1964.

In some situations, Title VII will allow discrimination on the part of the employer. These situations primarily encompass discriminating against a protected trait, most commonly sex, if an employer can suitably prove that the trait being discriminated against is a necessary (bona fide) occupational trait for the daily operation of the particular business in question. In order to use the bona fide occupational qualification defense and be permitted to discriminate, it is necessary for three traits to be shown: (1) There must be a direct relationship between the trait and the ability to perform the job; (2) the qualification must directly relate to the essence or central mission of the employer's business; and (3) there must also be no other alternative that is less restrictive or more reasonable.

Exhibit 5-2

Employers Who Fall Under the Auspices of the Civil Rights Act of 1964

- Private employers that have more than 15 employees
- Both public and private educational institutions
- State and local governments
- Public and private employment agencies
- Labor unions that have more than 15 members
- Labor management committees for apprenticeship and training

The exceptions that are allowed by the bona fide occupational qualification have been shown to exclude both religion (religion does not qualify, regardless of the position) and the preferences of customers or clientele of the business. Other situations that give carte blanche permission to an employer to forgo Title VII include dealing with an employee who is involved with the Communist party of the United States. Any of a multitude of other organizations that are required to list themselves with the federal government as a Communist-front or Communist-action group pursuant to the Subversive Activities Control Board final orders, resulting from the Subversive Activities Control Act of 1950, are also excluded from the Civil Rights Act protections. Partial and whole exceptions to the entirety of Title VII exist for Native American tribes, religious groups that perform work connected to the groups activities (including educational institutions), and bona fide nonprofit private member organizations. The federal government formerly had exemptions allocated to certain functions, but those have subsequently been removed (42 U.S.C. Section 2000e-16). Exhibit 5-3 lists employers excluded from the Civil Rights Act of 1964.

Exhibit 5-3

Employers Excluded from the Civil Rights Act of 1964

- Federally recognized Native American tribes
- Bona fide nonprofit membership organizations
- Religious groups that perform work directly related to the groups activities, including educational institutions

Strengthening the 1964 Legislation

Title VII is not the only antidiscrimination statute that governs employment law, nor has Title VII been without interpretation since its enactment. Both interpretation and subsequent amendment of the bill will be examined, though to facilitate discussion the original bill and its interpretation will be discussed first. The primary areas of interpretation of the original bill focus on the definitions attributed to sex discrimination.

The first cases involving sexual harassment as a form of discrimination began arising in the latter half of the 1970s. By the early 1980s, courts were consistently finding in favor of plaintiffs who filed suit against their employers for sexual discrimination arising from harassment. In 1986, the Supreme Court upheld sexual harassment as being discriminatory and thus protected under the auspices of Title VII. In 1998, the Supreme Court found that same-sex sexual harassment is possible. Based on its earlier decisions regarding sexual harassment as discrimination, the Court found that it too was protected by Title VII. Other findings of various courts and interpretations of legislators have led to supplemental bills that prohibit age discrimination, disability discrimination, and discrimination against pregnant women. To date, there has been no ruling on sexual orientation and cases of discrimination being protected under Title VII.

Augmenting the 1964 Legislation

The first piece of supplemental legislation that was passed to augment the Civil Rights Act of 1964 was the Age Discrimination in Employment Act (ADEA) of 1967. The ADEA expressly prohibits employment discrimination against people 40 years of age or older. Additionally, the ADEA defines standards for pensions and benefits that employers may provide along with requiring information regarding the unique needs of older workers be made public. In fact, the ADEA states that an employer (generally defined in much the same way as in Title VII) cannot "fail or refuse to hire or to discharge any individual or otherwise discriminate against any individual with respect to his compensation, terms, conditions, or privileges or employment, because of such individual's age." It is also unlawful for any employer to "limit, segregate, or classify his employees in any way which would deprive or tend to deprive any individual or employment opportunities or otherwise adversely affect his status as an employee, because of such individual's age." The ADEA does also note that it is against the law for any employer to cut the salary or wage rate of an employee in order to comply with the outlines of the ADEA. An exception to the age limits and discrimination is allowed in cases of mandatory retirement age for some occupations, primarily those that are executive level positions with a minimum yearly pension that exceeds a baseline. It is obvious to see the lineage of the ADEA, the verbiage used in the bill is virtually identical to that of the Civil Rights Act. One notable exception is that the ADEA applies to employers with 20 or more employees, while the Civil Rights Act requires a business to have only 15 employees.

Both the Civil Rights Act and the ADEA apply only to businesses involved in interstate commerce, regardless of size. Like the Title VII exclusions for bona fide occupational qualifications, such exclusions have been upheld by the ADEA. The exclusions for occupational qualifications are a bit broader with the ADEA. The exclusions range from the obvious (e.g., hiring a child to play the part of a child in a movie to the exclusion of older individuals) to instances where the safety of the public is in question (e.g., mandatory retirement ages for airline pilots). It should be noted that while the ADEA does prohibit discrimination and discriminatory preference against the young over the old, it does not prohibit favoring the old over the young. Particularly, what this means is that as an employee nears retirement, it is entirely appropriate for an employer to write benefit packages and engage in activities that favor them over younger employees (even if the younger employee is over 40 and ostensibly protected by the ADEA). This idea has been upheld in the court system, which has effectively negated claims of reverse age discrimination.

In 1972, Title VII of the Civil Rights Act of 1964 was officially amended for the first time. The amendment was inaugurated as the Equal Employment Opportunity Act of 1972. Specifically, the Equal Employment Act removed the protection of state and local governments (along with their employees) from antidiscrimination litigation. Prior to 1972, those individuals and agencies had been expressly excluded from the requirements of antidiscrimination hiring practices outlined in Title VII. Following the 1972 amendment, the only political exceptions were elected officials, their personal assistants, and their immediate advisors. Further, prior to 1972, the EEOC only had the ability to investigate and mediate probable cases, charges, and complaints brought under the auspices of Title VII; after 1972, they had the ability to bring suit on behalf of the plaintiffs.

The Equal Employment Opportunity Act made it unlawful for various conditions of employment such as wages to be extended based on the protected classes of Title VII, but it did allow exceptions to antidiscrimination charges when the discrimination was not based on a protected class. Therefore, it was thoroughly possible to discriminate against someone of a protected class *if* the discrimination was not based on their class, but on a nonassociated factor. For instance, it would be acceptable to discriminate against individuals relative to wage and pay-rate scales if the discrimination was based on merit, seniority, or quantity or quality of work, even if the individuals were in a protected class (once again, so long as the discrimination was not as a result of the protected class).

An important facet of the 1972 amendments to Title VII regarded recruiting and hiring employees. The Equal Employment Opportunity Act made it illegal for employers to utilize a method of recruiting or selecting members of their workforce (employees) that would either intentionally or *unintentionally* exclude or screen out minority group members. This has been interpreted to mean that certain recruiting tactics, such as "word-of-mouth" advertising, are expressly forbidden since they would by nature result in a nondiverse workforce. The government has found that word-of-mouth advertising does nothing more than perpetuate existing disparity (particularly racial disparity) in a workforce.

Quota hiring was expressly forbidden by the 1972 amendment. However, the law does note that disproportionate numbers of minority workers relative to geographical population makeup may be interpreted as discriminatory hiring. The government further notes that disproportionate minority group representation among subgroups of employees may also be deemed discriminatory (i.e., low numbers of minority supervisors). In the instances outlined previously, while quota hiring is expressly forbidden, the government would expect an employer to engage in targeted marketing to equalize the makeup of their workforce.

The 1972 Equal Employment Opportunity Act also generated the idea of disparate hiring requirements. The act included requirements for job listings that may identify the need for certain qualifications, thereby excluding groups of people are expressly forbidden. Unreasonably high standards for hire may be reason for the government to find that discriminatory practice exists; for instance, a height requirement, if not necessary to perform the job, may exclude females. Another example of expressly forbidden hiring practices includes having appearance or speech ability tests administered as a condition of employment since those may exclude members of certain minority groups. Photographs as a requirement to complete an application is expressly forbidden by the act.

The 1972 amendments also make unlawful, through further definition and clarification, sex discrimination. The act states it is unlawful for an employer to classify a job as "male" or "female." Policies that limit the employment of women in certain positions, or that require lifting a minimum weight that exceeds prescribed limits, or that exclude women for reasons of childbirth are unlawful under the authority of the 1972 act. It is also unlawful to initiate rules that limit or restrict the employment of either men or women as a result of their marital status. Any benefit an employer may grant that is contingent upon being the "head of household" or "principle wage earner" is forbidden by the amendments incorporated in the 1972 act.

Like all of the other bills, acts, and amendments, the Equal Employment Opportunity Act of 1972 allows for exceptions. One of the principle exclusions is for the bona fide occupational qualifications (e.g., hiring a female only to play a female role in a play). The 1972 act still excludes the wishes and preferences of clients, coworkers, employers, and customers as a viable reason for hiring an individual of one sex over another.

In 1978, the next supplement to Title VII was passed by the Congress, that is, the Pregnancy Discrimination Act (PDA). While both the original Civil Rights Act and the Equal Employment Opportunity Act of 1972 clarified and defined discrimination that resulted from sex, the acts only nominally addressed discrimination against gravid women. Like the previous amendments resulting in clarification of the 1964 act, the PDA qualifies discrimination that results from pregnancy, postpregnancy, or the ability to become pregnant as unlawful in companies that have more than 15 employees. Since the bill became active, employers are required by law to provide benefits (including leave pay, insurance, and support) to both women and men who are absent from work as a result of pregnancy or childbirth. Some states have taken this one step further and extended the benefit period to include time off for bonding with a new child (on the part of both parents, regardless of whether the child is biologically their own).

While the previous acts had numerous exclusions, perhaps the only viable exclusion to the PDA is when a company excludes pregnancy or childbirth as a viable excuse for missing work within a proscribed period following initial employment (e.g., women will not be allowed time off for childbirth until 1 full year of employment has been fulfilled). However to meet the mandates of the law and allow the exclusion, all medical conditions must be excluded in the same manner and the policy must apply equally to men and women. The law mandates that employers cannot institute mandatory childbirth leave times (i.e., employees must take 6 weeks off following the birth of their child), in addition to making it unlawful to force employees to take leave for childbirth or once a certain point has been reached (e.g., once the mother reaches 37 weeks of gestation, she is required to go on maternity leave). Essentially, the law holds that employees must be allowed to work as long as they desire and as long as they can fulfill the requirements of their position. It also holds that employees be allowed to return to their jobs (i.e., the job must be held open) as soon as they are willing and capable of fulfilling the requirements.

On July 26, 1990, George H. W. Bush signed into law the Americans with Disabilities Act of 1990 (ADA), which further strengthened the original 1964 Civil Rights Act. The bill was subsequently amended in 2008 (with the amendments taking effect on January 1, 2009). As discussed in previous chapters, the ADA legislation prohibits discrimination based on disability (under most circumstances).

The most recent large-scale update to the Civil Rights Act of 1964 is the Civil Rights Act of 1991. Enacted on November 21, 1991, the bill was specifically written to "amend the Civil Rights Act of 1964 to strengthen and improve federal civil rights laws, to provide for damages in cases of intentional employment discrimination, to clarify provisions regarding disparate impact actions, and for other purposes." The act was a direct counter to multiple challenges of the original Civil Rights Act in the US Supreme Court that had arisen after multiple groups of employees tried suing their employers for discrimination. The primary purposes of the act were to allow jury trials in discrimination cases, allow for damages as a result of emotional distress, and cap the amounts a jury could award in discrimination cases as monetary compensation for damages.

Like the 1964 act, the 1991 act is divided into titular sections. Title I of the 1991 act deals with Federal Civil Rights Remedies. Title II established a commission to study the artificial barriers to advancement of women and minorities in the work-place (a so-called "Glass Ceiling Commission"). Title III extended civil rights employment coverage to certain government employees. Title IV discusses the General Provisions Severability.

The first title prohibits racial discrimination in making and enforcing contracts, including employment contracts. It also allocates specific damages in cases of intentional discrimination; in effect, Title I sets limits on damages that may be received in cases arising from discrimination, including the awarding of attorney's fees for the winner of suits. Title I also expressly prohibits the use of test scores in discriminatory fashion. Title I also allows an employer to use as a defense in discrimination cases the fact (upon proof) that the decision reached between themselves and the employee would have been the same regardless of the employees status as a protected minority. This defense relieves the employer of any mandate to reimburse back pay or to reinstate the employee if it can be shown that the individual's status as a minority had nothing to do with the decision that was reached, even if the employee can show discrimination. However, the defense does not relieve liability for legal fees that may have been incurred, even though no other damages may be awarded.

Title II of the 1991 act established a "Glass Ceiling Commission" that was explicitly tasked with completing a study that examined "artificial barriers to the advancement of women and minorities in the workplace." Further, the commission was tasked with making whatever recommendations it felt were warranted to overcome the barriers it had identified. It is important to note that this commission was separate from the EEOC.

Title III extended the coverage and protection guaranteed by the 1964 Civil Rights Act to employees of the government who had been previously exempt from liability. State governments were now subject to the provisions of anti-discrimination law and could not use race, color, religion, sex, national origin, age, or disability to exclude anyone from the benefits of state employment. Also included for the first time were individuals who had been previously expressly denied antidiscrimination protection (in the Civil Rights Act of 1964). Individuals who were appointed to be members of an elected official's personal staff, excluded under the Civil Rights Act of 1964, were now extended coverage under the Civil Rights Act of 1991.

The fourth and final title of the 1991 is exclusively a severability clause. The General Provisions Severability clause states that if any portion of the act is found to be invalid, then the remainder of the act shall exist unto itself. Therefore, each portion of the act would be treated separately if one title or statement was found to be unsound, it would be the only thing affected.

Perhaps the most important aspect of the 1991 act was the ability of an employer to be found guilty of "unintentional discrimination." Unintentional discrimination exists when there are disparate numbers (based on statistical analysis) of minorities in the employers workforce compared with the pool of prospective employees (the population) from which they are drawn. Effectively what that means is that if an employer subjectively evaluates qualifications in order to determine employment eligibility, and if subsequent analysis shows that there are fewer minorities than are found in the general population from which the employers workforce is drawn, then the employers hiring process is discriminatory.

John Cook most clearly enumerates the ways an employer can protect itself from unintentional discrimination in his 1992 article in *Labor Management Decisions*. In the article, Cook notes that "there are several practical and fairly easy steps that employers can implement . . . that will make a world of difference . . . if an allegation of unintentional discrimination emerges." The steps are as follows:

1. *Collect and maintain applicant flow data.* The collection of data is integral to a defense of an employer's hiring decisions. The burden of proof falls to the employer to show that the applicants are indicative of the hiring pool and not an aberrance that results in discrimination or the favoring of one group of applicants over another. If the employer is incapable of demonstrating the applicant pool, it is possible for the plaintiff to use general workforce statistics and the assumption will be that applicants were representative of each demographic group found in the population regardless of whether or not this is the case. It is important to note, that while data should be collected that relates to a prospective employee's sex, race, color, national origin, and age to demonstrate (should the need arise) the pool of prospective employees, this information must be kept separate from data used to actually select employees. Further, individuals involved in making employment decisions cannot legally have access to applicants' demographic data.

2. *Limit the pool of applicants.* It is important to realize that applicant pools must be minimized to reduce the risk of statistical litigation. If this reduction in the applicant pool is not undertaken, the law will make the assumption that everyone that completed an application was qualified and considered for every single job open or listed during a period of time. To circumvent this potential issue, employers can limit the length of time an application will be considered "active" (e.g., stating that applications will only be considered for positions that are open within 30 days of the applications filing). Do not accept unsolicited applications. Discard any application that is illegible or incomplete. Finally, accept applications only when a job is open and being filled. Do not maintain a file of prospective applicants.

3. *Use written job descriptions.* This is perhaps the most commonsense item; however, it is often underutilized. Each job description should identify the specific duties and qualifications required for a job. However, the employer should be capable of defending the qualifications they enumerate as being

valid predictors of job performance. The more clearly stated hiring criteria are, the less likely an employer will be to face discrimination proceedings.

4. *Post promotional opportunities.* Cook implicitly states that claims of unintentional discrimination commonly arise from instances in which promotions are arbitrarily announced without being posted. By posting specific criteria for promotion and an application deadline, the employer can protect itself from being sued by identifying the pool of candidates before the choice is made.

5. *Use objective screening criteria at an early stage.* Generally, employment decisions are arrived at through a process of elimination. The earlier in the process that objective elimination occurs the sooner unqualified candidates can be identified and removed from the prospective pool of applicants. Again, it is important to justify the criteria used to eliminate the candidate and correlate it directly to their prospective job performance.

6. *Maintain records of employment decisions.* This is perhaps the most important step for employers to undertake in trying to avoid unintentional discrimination cases. Since the law can shift the burden of proof to an employer in discrimination cases (it is the employer's responsibility to show there was no discrimination versus the plaintiffs responsibility to show that the employer did discriminate), it is incumbent upon the employer to show that decisions relevant to employment were objective and that they were legitimately made based on job-related qualifications and not on protected demographic categories. See Exhibit 5-4 for a listing of ways of avoiding unintentional discrimination.

Exhibit 5-4

Ways to Avoid Cases of Unintentional Discrimination According to John Cook

- Collect and maintain applicant flow data.
- Limit the pool of applicants.
- Use written job descriptions.
- Post promotional opportunities.
- Use objective screening criteria at an early stage.
- Maintain records of employment decisions.

Source: Cook (1992)

Enforcement

It is the primary responsibility of the US Equal Employment Opportunity Commission (EEOC) to enforce all of the antidiscrimination laws in America against private employers. It also falls to the EEOC to provide governmental oversight (and by association, coordination) of all the federal employment regulations, practices, or policies. Enforcement of Title VII against governmental agencies, both state and federal, falls to the Employment Litigation Section, Civil Rights Division of the US Department of Justice. Regardless of who is responsible for enforcement, either the EEOC or the Employment Litigation Section, any employee who feels he or she has been unfairly discriminated against or has been the victim of any type of discriminatory act by an employer is required to file a charge of discrimination with the EEOC within 180 days of the alleged act. Therefore, regardless of who the enforcing agent will be, the EEOC processes all claims and charges of discrimination that allege a violation of Title VII.

Exceptions to the 180 day filing limit do exist and include individuals who may have filed charges with a state agency, or individuals who reside in a state that has an antidiscrimination enforcement agency (regardless of whether or not a complaint is filed with that agency); in each of these cases, the plaintiff has 300 days to file a complaint with the EEOC. These Fair Employment Practices Agencies (FEPAs) exist to aid the EEOC in investigating, mediating, and filing lawsuits on behalf of employees who feel they have been discriminated against. Arkansas and Alabama are currently the only two states that do not have FEPAs.

Conclusion

The Civil Rights Act of 1964, along with subsequent reinforcements through amendment (particularly in 1991) has, in theory, leveled the workplace playing field. While full parity has yet to be found across all working classes and groups, the legislation has worked to ensure nominal equality and remove intentional discrimination against employees on the part of their employers. Title VII of the act particularly prohibits discrimination based on race, color, religion, sex, or national origin in employment. The probability that an employer will face trouble resulting from a discrimination suit is increasingly high; as a result, effective legal counsel for the employer is absolutely imperative. However, working knowledge of the mandates of the law should allow a manager to remain relatively faultless in any litigation that may arise.

Questions for Review and Discussion

1. What, primarily, did the Civil Rights Act of 1991 add to the provisions of Title VII of the Civil Rights Act of 1964?
2. What are disparate hiring requirements and of what may they consist?

3. What caused the Civil Rights Act of 1875 to fail? Explain.

4. In what ways did the Equal Employment Act affect Title VII?

5. Define protected classes, and describe as many as you can think of.

6. Explain the intended purpose of collecting applicant flow data in the recruitment and employment process.

7. Cite and explain at least three instances in which gender or age may be considered a bona fide occupational qualification.

8. Explain why sexual harassment is legally considered a form of sex discrimination.

9. Explain the apparent intent of the Glass Ceiling Commission and identify the authority under which it was to function.

10. In what significant way did the Age Discrimination in Employment Act add to age-discrimination protection as provided under Title VII?

Bibliography

Acemoglu, D., & Angrist, J. D. (2001). Consequences of employment protection? The case of the Americans with Disabilities Act. *Journal of Political Economy, 109,* 915–957.

Age Discrimination in Employment Act. Pub.L. 90–202, 81 Stat. 602 (1967, December 15).

Americans with Disabilities Act. Pub.L. 101–336, 104 Stat. 327 (1990, July 26).

Ashbrook Center for Public Affairs. (2006). *The Civil Rights Act of 1866.* Available at: http://teachingamericanhistory.org/library/index.asp?document-480. Accessed May 26, 2010.

Ashbrook Center for Public Affairs. (2006). *The Civil Rights Act of 1875.* Available at: http://teachingamericanhistory.org/library/index.asp?document-481. Accessed May 26, 2010.

Branch, T. (1999). *Pillar of fire: America in the King years 1963–1965.* New York: Simon and Schuster.

Burstein, P. (1985). *Discrimination, jobs and politics: The struggle for equal employment opportunity in the United States since the New Deal.* Chicago: University of Chicago Press.

Center for American Progress. (2004, July 2). *The Civil Rights Act 40 years later.* Available at: http://www.americanprogress.org/issues/2004/07/b106855.html/print.html. Accessed May 26, 2010.

Civil Rights Act of 1866, 14 Stat. 27 (1866).

Civil Rights Act of 1870 (The Enforcement Act), 16 Stat. 140 (1870).

Civil Rights Act of 1871, 17 Stat. 13 (1871).

Civil Rights Act of 1875, 18 Stat. 335 (1875).

Civil Rights Act of 1964. Pub.L. 88–352, 78 Stat. 241 (1964, July 2).

Civil Rights Act of 1991, Pub.L. 102–166 (1991, November 21).

Cook, J. C. (1992). Prepare to avoid trouble under the Civil Rights Act of 1991 [Electronic version]. *Labor Management Decisions, 2*(2). Available at: http://apmp.berkeley.edu/APMP/pubs/lmd/html/summer_92/preparetoav.html. Accessed May 26, 2010.

Culp, J. M. (1986). Federal courts and the enforcement of Title VII. *AEA Papers and Proceedings, 76*(2), 355–358.

Developments in the law—Employment discrimination and Title VII of the Civil Rights Act of 1964. (1971). *Harvard Law Review, 84,* 1109–1316.

Dirksen Congressional Center. (2006). *Major features of the Civil Rights Act of 1964.* Available at: http://www.congresslink.org/print_basics_histmats_civilrights64text.htm. Accessed May 26, 2010.

Finley, K. M. (2008). *Delaying the dream: Southern Senators and the fight against civil rights, 1938–1965.* Baton Rouge, LA: LSU Press.

Freeman, J. (1991). How "sex" got into Title VII: Persistent opportunism as a maker of public policy. *Law and Inequality: A Journal of Theory and Practice, 9*(2), 163–184.

Graham, H. (1990). *The Civil Rights Era: Origins and development of national policy, 1960–1972.* New York: Oxford University Press.

Loevy, R. D. (n.d.). *A brief history of The Civil Rights Act of 1964.* Available at: http://faculty1.coloradocollege.edu/bloevy/civilrightsactof1964. Accessed May 26, 2010.

Loevy, R. D. (1997). *The Civil Rights Act of 1964: The passage of the law that ended racial segregation.* New York: State University of New York.

National Archives. (n.d.). *Teaching with documents: The Civil Rights Act of 1964 and the Equal Employment Opportunity Commission.* Available at: http://www.archives.gov/education/lessons/civil-rights-act/. Accessed May 26, 2010. 1866 Civil Rights Act 14 Stat. 27–30 (1866, April 9).

Nowicki, M., & Summers, J. (2006, April). Poor management can look like discrimination. *Healthcare Financial Management, 60*(4), 118–119.

O'Brien, R. (Ed.) (2004). *Voices from the edge: Narratives about the Americans With Disabilities Act.* New York: Oxford University Press.

Piar, D. F. (2001). The uncertain future of Title VII class actions after the Civil Rights Act of 1991. *Brigham Young University Law Review,* 305–347.

Robinson, R. K., Franklin, G. M., Tinney, C. H., Crow, S. M., & Hartman, S. J. (2005). Sexual harassment in the workplace: Guidelines for educating healthcare managers. *Journal of Health and Human Services Administration, 27*(4), 501–530.

Rosenbaum, S., Markus, A., & Darnell, J. (2000). U.S. civil rights policy and access to health care by minority Americans: Implications for a changing health care system. *Medical Care Research and Review, 57*(Suppl. 1), 236–259.

Switzer, J. V. (2003). *Disabled rights: American disability policy and the fight for equality.* Washington, DC: Georgetown University Press.

US Department of State. (2009). *Free at last: The U.S. civil rights movement.* Available at: http://www.america.gov/publications/books-content/free-at-last.pdf. Accessed May 26, 2010.

US Department of Justice, Civil Rights Division. (2009). *Employment litigation section frequently asked questions.* Available at: http://www.usdoj.gov/crt/emp/faq.php. Accessed May 26, 2010.

US Equal Employment Opportunity Commission. (1978). *Facts about pregnancy discrimination.* Available at: http://www.eeoc.gov/facts/fs-preg.html. Accessed May 26, 2010.

US Equal Employment Opportunity Commission. (1990). *Disability discrimination.* Available at: http://www.eeoc.gov/laws/types/disability.cfm. Accessed May 26, 2010.

US Equal Employment Opportunity Commission. (2009). *Federal laws prohibiting job discrimination questions and answers.* Available at: http://www.eeoc.gov/facts/qanda.html. Accessed May 26, 2010.

US Senate. (n.d.). *June 10, 1964, civil rights filibuster ended.* Available at: http://www.senate.gov/artandhistory/history/minute/Civil_Rights_Filibuster_Ended.htm. Accessed May 26, 2010.

Whalen, C., & Whalen, B. (1985). *The longest debate: A legislative history of the 1964 Civil Rights Act.* Cabin John, MD: Seven Locks Press.

Chapter 6

Interviewing and Reference Checking

Carol A. Campbell, DBA, RHIA, FAHIMA, *Professor, Health Informatics, Medical College of Georgia, Augusta, Georgia*

Chapter Objectives

- Introduce the concepts of the job analysis and the job description and describe how they apply as prerequisite to preparation for an effective employee placement interview.
- Review the principal laws relevant to recruiting and interviewing, and discuss their implications for interview conduct.
- Identify several kinds of questions that are illegal in the employment interview process.
- Review the different types of interviews and establish which types are best employed in what kinds of interview situations.
- Provide a number of specific tips for the conduct of a successful and legal employment interview.
- Examine different approaches for checking employment references and how to avoid related problems.

Introduction

Hiring the right person requires you to know yourself, know the applicable law, and be trustful but prepared to verify all pertinent information. Knowing yourself—that is, knowing your business—allows you to begin with an objective in mind. Knowing the law allows you to reach your objective without unnecessary or unpleasant detours. A properly conducted interview is a search for a measure of agreement between interviewer and applicant; reference checking, which follows, is the process of verifying the "truth" as set forth by the applicant.

Interviews, whether experienced as an interviewee or interviewer, are often looked upon as a less than pleasant experience that one might just as soon avoid. The Merriam-Webster's online thesaurus provided the following response to the word *interview*: "The word you've entered isn't in the thesaurus."[1] None of the other words suggested by the thesaurus lead us to a useful description of the employment interview process.

A brief survey of references on the legal aspects of interviewing may cause many to conclude that the hiring process is a tangled mass of confusing employment laws.

The goal of this chapter is to leave the reader with a positive outlook on the kinds of interactions labeled as interviews. Some reassurance can be found in the simple observation that the ability to carry on a conversation is evidence that one has the ability to succeed on either side of an interview. The most successful conversationalists share a common trait: They know themselves, and that knowledge frees them to focus on the needs, interests, and responses of the other party to the conversation. This rationale extends to the context of job interviews. This chapter addresses the steps necessary to ensure a successful interview conversation from the perspective of an employer seeking to fill a vacant position.

Know Yourself

Hire someone you can live with. After all, in practical terms, that is what will happen after the hiring. This is not at all to suggest that the entire web of employment laws can be completely disregarded. Rather, it is to point out that, in reality, employers do have great leeway in making employment decisions. To the dismay of a great many job applicants, employers even have the leeway to hire on the basis of favoritism, revenge, random or erroneous judgment, illogicality, mere error, or any other reason except intentional discrimination.[2] Of course, taking leeway to such extremes will likely result in applicants filing complaints typically citing violations of the Civil Rights Act of 1964 as presented in Chapter 5. With the extreme possibilities noted, a closer look at an ethical application of knowing yourself is in order.

Matching a person to a position is the end goal of the interviewing and hiring process. The ability to know when the right person has been identified requires knowing the employment context from both a macro and micro view. For example, the macro view involves knowing the following:

- The purpose and mission of the business organization—is it service or production?
- The geographical range of the business—is it local, state, national, or international?

- The specifics of the opening within the organization—is it in operations or administration? Is it junior or senior level?

A micro view involves knowledge of the specifics of the position:

- What are the overall job duties?
- What are the essential or primary duties?
- What are the secondary or peripheral duties?
- To whom does this position report? And who, if anyone, reports to this position?
- What are the necessary educational requirements of the position?
- What prior work experiences are necessary or desirable for the position?
- What personal qualifications and skills are required for the position?

The best way to answer these and other job-related questions is to conduct a thorough *job analysis*. The job analysis is a systematic means of identifying and assessing detailed information about a job. Systematic job analysis results in knowledge of the duties, tasks, and activities required of the job holder. This provides the employer with everything required to develop a new job description or revise an existing job description.

The *job description* is an important document that serves multiple purposes, including serving as a guide to job recruitment postings or advertisements. Note that the terms *job* and *position*, while used interchangeably in casual conversation, often differ in meaning. A job is a group of activities and duties that comprise units of work. A position consists of units of work assigned to and performed by one specific person. To illustrate, consider a healthcare facility that employs 10 occupational therapists, filling 10 positions. These occupational therapists all perform the same job, but they are assigned to 10 separate positions.

The micro view of a job, as previously noted, is captured in a written job description. There is no universal job description format used by all organizations, but a few essential elements must be present in a well-structured job description. The job description elements should include:

- Clear identification of the job;
- A summary of the job's purposes—why it exists and what it is intended to accomplish;
- Enumeration of the job duties; and
- The qualifications of persons who will perform this job.

The *identification* section typically includes the job title, job code, department or unit, and title of the immediate supervisor. A picture may be worth a thousand words, and a well-thought-out job title presents a fairly complete "picture" of the job in a few precise terms. *The Dictionary of Occupational Titles (DOT), Fourth Edition*, created by the US Employment Service in 1939 and last updated in 1991, is a useful tool in the development of job descriptions and job titles. (This guide is available online at: http://www.oalj.dol.gov/libdot.htm)

The *job summary* section is precisely that, a brief narrative picture of the job. This section usually appears immediately below the identification section, consequently the reader can quickly see what the job entails first from the title and then by reading what is essentially an expanded version of the title in the summary section. Again, the *DOT* may be a useful guide in developing this section.

The *duties* section is the most common part of job descriptions. This section describes, usually in a numbered outline format, the major duties and responsibilities of the job holder. This section is not intended to be an all-inclusive. Frankly, for many jobs, complete inclusiveness of all likely tasks is nearly impossible. Rather, the duties section should describe the essential job duties, those regular or routine duties that comprise most of the job. For most jobs, a fairly complete description of duties can usually be provided in about 10 (and occasionally fewer) statements. Present tense and action verbs should be employed in writing concise and to-the-point job duty statements. Another indication of a well-written job description is a limited number of pages. Much like employment resumes, a well-written job description can usually fit on one or two pages.[3]

The minimum qualifications a person must posses to be considered for hire (and for successful job performance thereafter) are provided in the qualifications section. This part of the job description is also referred to as the person or employee-specification section. Minimum requirements for education, training, and prior experience are described in this section. Employers need to be careful to avoid confusing this section with another common section referred to as *job specifications*. The minimum person or employee specifications or qualifications are used to aid employers in selecting the right person for the job. On the other hand, job specifications are used for wage and salary determination purposes through a process commonly referred to *job evaluation*, by which a job's classification and pay grade are determined. A complete discussion of job evaluation is beyond the scope of this chapter; however, the specifications developed using this process describe the job in terms of compensable factors. Four broad categories are used: skill, effort, responsibility, and working conditions. These may be further subdivided into more refined factors (e.g., effort may be divided into the physical and mental effort required to do the job).

Know the Law

One need not be a lawyer to know enough employment law to steer clear of legal trouble.

With a job description in hand, the employer is equipped with knowledge of the questions that should be asked of applicants. One goal of an employee selection interview is to be as consistent and objective as possible. Using the job description as the primary reference point is the best way to ensure objectivity, consistency, and compatibility with legal requirements. As previously suggested, employers have considerable leeway in what they can ask of an applicant. The precaution in present-day interview questioning is the essential avoidance of all questions that can be construed as discriminatory. Questions that could be perceived as discriminating against "protected classes," as defined by federal legislation (primarily Title VII of the Civil Rights Act of 1964). Sticking to strictly job-related questions, with total emphasis on what the individual *knows*, *has done*, and *can do*, and complete avoidance of questions of a personal nature, is the surest way to both identifying the most qualified applicant and avoiding legal complaints.

The key federal laws that employers should keep well in mind when formulating nondiscriminatory interview questions include the Civil Rights Act of 1964 and its amendments (see Chapter 5); the Americans with Disabilities Act (see Chapter 4); and the Age Discrimination in Employment Act (ADEA) of 1967 and its amendments. These laws prohibit discriminatory employment practices throughout all phases of recruitment, interviewing, hiring, and placement on the basis of race, color, religion, national origin, gender, disability, or age. The provisions of these laws make it illegal to ask job applicants questions in the following categories before hiring: marital status, height and weight, number and ages of dependents, information about spouse, age-related questions, health status, arrests, religious affiliation, and native tongue or language used at home. Examples of inappropriate or illegal questions include inquires such as:

- Are you married? (Any question that asks about the existence of a spouse, or that can be construed as fishing for such information is forbidden.)
- Have you any dependents? (A similarly forbidden question. Some employers attempt to avoid hiring single parents under the assumption that such employees have more attendance problems than others.)
- How old are you? or What is your date of birth? (The only legal question that can be asked about age is: Are you at least 18 years of age? This is applicable because of various states' child labor laws governing the employment of persons younger than age 18. The only other exceptions are those few instances in which age can be considered a bona fide occupational qualification [BFOQ]).
- How tall are you? How much do you weigh? (Again, personal information that is irrelevant in the hiring process. There have been legal challenges by individuals who claim to have been rejected for employment because of being "too heavy.")
- When did you graduate from high school or college? (Questions involving dates other than dates of employment can be construed as fishing for indications of age.)
- Have you ever been arrested? (You may ask about *convictions* but not arrests. An arrest in and of itself embodies an allegation that may or may not be proven.)

- What organizations do you belong to? (This question must be limited to work-related organizations only, such as professional societies. The names of many other kinds of organizations identify or imply certain personal information such as ethnicity or religion.)
- Who should we contact in case of emergency and what is your relationship to this person? (Again, a question that can be seen as fishing for family status.)
- What is the origin of your name? From where did your parents come? (Any question concerning national, ethnic, or racial origin is forbidden.)
- What is your gender? (Although usually obvious, this cannot be directly asked.)
- Have you ever filed a Workers' Compensation claim? (Illegal inquiry seen as attempting to determine whether an applicant might represent a risk of future such claims.)
- What is the nature of any illness or physical limitation you have had or currently have? (This is fishing for indications of real or potential disability. The only safe questions in this realm are on the order of: Do you have any condition that could limit your ability to properly perform the major functions of this job?)
- Are you or have you ever been a member of a labor union? (This is forbidden because of an assumed tendency for employers to avoid persons who might opt for union organizing.)

Generally, the foregoing and similar questions are considered inappropriate pre-hire inquiries because they ask for characteristics of applicants, which, if known by the employer, can be construed as reasons for rejecting applicants for employment. None of the elements of forbidden information—essentially, personal information—can legally be used as the basis for rejecting an individual for employment. Thus, if the employer has such knowledge of personal information and an applicant is rejected, the applicant can claim to have been turned down for discriminatory reasons. Even if an applicant volunteers personal information (e.g., "I'm a single parent and I really need a job."), the hiring manager cannot be influenced by this in making a hiring decision. (One particular kind of problem that can make interviewing treacherous at times is the occasional applicant who will attempt to "trap" the interviewer by volunteering personal information so as to later claim rejection on the basis of that information.)

Some questions that are inappropriate before hiring are necessary and legal after an applicant has accepted an offer of employment. For example, most employers have a legitimate need for emergency contact information as well as personal information necessary for employee benefits purposes. Also, many employers retain demographic information regarding applicants, interviewees, and hires that may be required for Affirmative Action and other legal purposes.

Necessary personal information must always be collected after hire. One convenient method involves designing the application form with a tear off portion to keep separate from the information seen by the interviewer. A 2005 study of litigation commonly associated with application forms found the issues primarily involve inappropriate questions about the gender and age of applicants.[4]

EEOC and Uniform Guidelines

As discussed in Chapter 5, Title VII of the Civil Rights Act of 1964 established the Equal Employment Opportunity Commission (EEOC) to enforce the provisions of the act. The 1978 Uniform Guidelines on Employee Selection Procedures are regulations published by the EEOC and other federal agencies associated with fair employment. These guidelines apply to all employer procedures used to select, promote, transfer, demote, dismiss, and refer applicants and employees. The guidelines provide employers with explanations and interpretations of federal fair employment laws. If actions by the employer have a disproportionate effect (disparate treatment or impact) on a protected class, the employer will be required to prove a business necessity for this outcome. The Uniform Guidelines describe the various methods employers can use to demonstrate that a particular selection method or job requirement is necessary. If the employer is unable to satisfactorily prove business necessity, the employer will be required to change procedures to eliminate the impact. Discrimination lawsuits based on disparate impact can be brought by applicants affected by nonvalidated hiring procedures.[5]

Business necessity and *job relatedness* are terms of law associated with the application of the Uniform Guidelines. Policies, procedures, and practices necessary for business efficiency, effectiveness, and safety are a business necessity. This is also an area that has kept the courts busy. Employers frequently identify minimum levels of education as required for successful performance on the job, and this requirement emerges in the screening of applicants. For example, if an employer requires a high school diploma as the minimum education qualification for applicants and new hires, the employer must be able to defend the requirement as essential to the successful performance of the job. Although most jobs do require employees to at least have minimal skill in reading or math, requiring a high school diploma as evidence that this skill level is met can likely be questioned by the EEOC. In recruiting for entry-level positions, some employers successfully avoid the implied trap by asking not for a high school diploma, but rather for the "ability to read and write and follow simple instructions." Whatever minimum requirements are set by the employer, it is critical that the employer be able to prove the requirement is directly job related.

It is not illegal for requirements to have a greater impact on protected classes, but the requirements must not be established for purposes of deliberately screening out minorities and women. However, the 1971 landmark case of *Griggs v. Duke Power* makes it clear that lack of discriminatory intent is not enough for validating employment practices. The employer has the burden of proof to demonstrate that employment requirements are directly job related as a business necessity. For example, in the *Griggs v. Duke Power* case, the US Supreme Court ruled the employer's requirement for a minimum score on an intelligence test and a high school diploma were not job related and were therefore discriminatory in that particular employment situation.[6]

An exception to Title VII of the 1964 Civil Rights Act is the employer's right to discriminate on the basis of gender, religion, or national origin if the required characteristic is a BFOQ. Consequently, employers can exclude persons from consideration for interviews or hiring for reasons that would otherwise be illegal. What qualifies as a legitimate BFOQ has been addressed by courts throughout the United States; as a result, there are a variety of interpretations. Examples include court decisions that deem it legal for Chinese restaurant employers to hire only Asians to serve customers and for Catholic churches to only hire Catholics for certain positions in those churches. There is limited justification for age as a BFOQ; generally, the legal exception consists of jobs for which the safety of the public is central. Thus, some courts have ruled that for the jobs of police officers, firefighters, and airline pilots age is a BFOQ.[7]

Interview Styles

There are two broad categories of interview style: structured and unstructured (or at least less structured). As these terms more than imply, the primary difference between categories is the degree to which the interview questions are predetermined and how closely the interviewer follows a "script." The more structured the interview, the more rigid it is in terms of sticking with a prescribed list of questions.

Highly structured interviews involve asking closed-ended questions (i.e., those that elicit a simple brief response). In practice, employers frequently use both interview styles. Initial screening of applicants may be handled through structured interviews conducted by human resources to determine whether applicants possess the minimum qualifications needed, and those applicants who "make the cut" are then scheduled for a second round of less-structured interviews. Sometimes employers apply different styles depending on the type and number of positions to be filled. Entry-level positions are frequently filled following a process of structured interviews, the goal of which is to simply identify individuals who meet the minimum qualifications for jobs that have limited advancement potential. If a large number of positions need to be filled, this approach is efficient and usually effective. Examples of structured interview questions include:

- What position are you applying for?
- Can you work the job's specified hours?
- Do you have the legal right to work in the United States?
- Are you at least 18 years of age?
- What training or education qualifies you for this job?

- What qualities do you posses that qualify you for this position?
- What is your past work experience?

For a vacant position at a higher level that includes responsibilities for managing people and other resources, employers typically probe deeper through a process of less-structured or unstructured interviews. The interview may begin with a standard set of questions, perhaps asking applicants to describe their behavioral tendencies when faced with difficult situations. This kind of interview is best accomplished by asking more free-flowing or open-ended questions. In fact, this interview approach is variously referred to as behavioral interviewing or situational interviewing.

There is a practical limit to the extent to which questions should be open ended. The best questions require the applicant to supply an answer in a few sentences, continuing to speak with the interviewer in a conversational style. Even an open-ended question must give the interviewee some boundaries within which to respond. The less-structured questions supplied in the list that follows are good examples. The open-ended question that provides no boundaries should be avoided. One such question—actually more of a command than a question—sometimes used by un-skilled or ill-prepared interviewers to open the interview is "Tell me about yourself." This is grossly unfair to the applicant, who is given no idea of where to start, how much to say, or what is really wanted.

An extreme approach to the situational interview is the "stress interview" in which the interviewer attempts to deliberately pressure an applicant and create anxiety for the purpose of assessing how the person deals with high-stress situations. This approach has drawbacks, not the least of which is the risk of applicants forming a negative view of the employer and thus turning down job offers. Since qualified employees can be difficult to find, playing the role of an obnoxious interviewer may be unwise.

A few examples of less-structured interview questions follow:

- Why did you leave your most recent job, or why are you planning on leaving your current position?
- Describe what you consider to be ideal job.
- What type of responsibilities do you find most rewarding?
- What type of responsibilities do you find frustrating?
- How do you go about forming good relationships with coworkers?
- Describe a "crisis" situation you experienced and how you handled it. What were the results?
- Describe three tough decisions you made in the last year. What made these decisions difficult? What alternatives did you consider? Describe the end results. What would you do differently if given the opportunity to relive the experience?
- Describe an accomplishment you are proud of.

- Describe an area of your performance you are dissatisfied with. How would your current or past supervisor answer this question about you?
- Describe accomplishments that you initiated (outside your "typical" job expectations) that benefited your current or past employer.

Follow-up questions that probe deeper include asking candidates to explain, for example:

- Exactly how were you involved in this particular situation?
- What actions did you take and what were the specific results?
- Describe the relationships among others involved and the help you may have received from them.
- Under what certain conditions were the resulting actions taken, and how might these conditions have influenced the choices made?

Tips for Successful Interviewing

1. Be prepared. An interview is never the time to "wing it" or play it off the cuff. Thoroughly review the job description in advance of the interview. Know the responsibilities and the minimum qualifications required for successful job performance.
2. Determine the interview style that best suits the particular job selection scenario, and develop a list of questions accordingly.
3. Choose an interview environment free of other distractions and interruptions. Absolute privacy is essential.
4. Set aside adequate time for the interview. All the preparation in the world may be useless if the interview is rushed.
5. Allow the applicant to ask questions. The thorough interview is a conversation.
6. Avoid reaching premature conclusions about the applicant. Finish the interview and assess the results before making up your mind.
7. If the applicant is coming across as perfect or nearly so, adjust your line of questioning to dig deeper or look for inconsistencies. One who quickly comes across as too good to be true is often just that.
8. Avoid asking leading questions, those that essentially give the applicant the answers you want to hear. This is a particular danger with an applicant who is quickly shaping up favorably in your mind.
9. Do more listening and less talking in the interview conversation. You cannot learn about an applicant by talking about yourself or your organization.
10. Take notes. Do very little writing while conversing; you cannot write and listen effectively at the same time. Write down your impressions and conclusions immediately after the interview.

Trust but Verify

Although skilled interviewers can and should trust their instincts after interviewing applicants, the adage "trust but verify" applies to making the right selection. The step of reference checking is essential to ensure that unqualified applicants or those with criminal records are not hired for positions for which they are unsuited.

Reference checking poses some problems for employers. Employers are caught between two legal risks: complaints by former employees and complaints by the new employers or their employees. Former employees have successfully sued past employers for defamation based on negative responses to inquiries from potential employers. Hiring an unfit employee, particularly one with a history of violence, leaves the new employer open for charges of negligent hiring if the person commits a similar act.[8]

Courts have found past employers guilty of defamation, slander, libel, or retaliatory violation of Title VII for providing negative references that are false, unfounded, or misleading. Concern over lawsuits by former employees has influenced employers to either decline requests for references or at least significantly limit the information provided in response to an inquiry by a potential employer. However, a refusal to provide a reference may also bring about a claim of retaliation by a former employee. Consequently, many employers will provide only verification of employment and relevant dates, a description of the position held, and salary range.

Risk to a previous employer increases if the applicant left the position via involuntary termination. Generally, this risk can be minimized by stating only the verifiable facts associated with the applicant's departure and avoiding editorializing. Speculation, subjective assessments, personality judgments, and opinion can cause problems. A truthful statement, made in response to a direct question and verifiable in an official record, is the only appropriate response. Employers are afforded some protection when divulging factual negative information without malicious intent. The doctrine of qualified privilege protects employers who, in good faith, provide accurate yet negative information about a former employee to a potential employer.

Failure to either check references or to adequately probe for relevant information about an applicant may result in claims of negligent hiring. Such cases often arise when a new employer should have known or could have known significant facts about the applicant but as a consequence of not checking references hired an unsuitable person. More specifically, these cases ordinarily involve the hiring of individuals who have committed violence in their previous positions and then committed the same or similar acts at their new jobs.

There is another fundamental reason for checking references: People lie. Sometimes they lie knowingly, sometimes they lie by omission, and sometimes they bend the truth and try to put something questionable in a favorable light. Resume fraud is an ever-present problem. Claims regarding career accomplishments and education that are either exaggerated or entirely false appear on resumes all too frequently. When employment markets tighten, the storytelling by applicants usually increases.

Potential employers should carefully check academic and training credentials of applicants as well as information offered about prior positions.

Applicants may sometimes "forget" to include key terms in their prior titles that would reveal their responsibilities were not as significant as they may wish the potential employer to believe. Terms such as "junior" or "assistant" give an entirely different meaning to job titles. A different employment picture also can be painted by the manner in which employment dates are reported. Applicants who have a sketchy or fragmented job history may attempt to mask this reality by only listing the years of employment. For example, there is a big difference between the implication of an employment time frame listed as 2007–2009 (which appears to be 2 full years) and the realities of actual employment from December 15, 2007 to January 2, 2009 (barely more than 1 year). Also, significant gaps in an applicant's experience call for closer questioning to determine whether anything potentially unflattering has been omitted.

Some employers attempt to evaluate an applicant's level of responsibility by checking credit history. Theory suggests that a responsible person will have a good credit record and vice versa. This approach to applicant assessment makes sense for positions in which incumbents will have access to or responsibility for money, but employers that check credit histories must comply with the federal Fair Credit Reporting Act. Compliance with the act requires that the employer obtain the consent of the applicant and furnish the applicant with a copy of the report. State law should also be consulted as these laws may limit or prohibit credit checks. Also, the EEOC has determined that unnecessary credit checks may be illegal in some cases. Generally, these cases are associated with disparate impact.[9]

Other challenges in reference checking involve oral versus written requests and oral versus written responses. These challenges are connected to the issues of potential claims of defamation and negligent hiring. Naturally, potential employers prefer written responses, whereas many former employers would rather provide oral responses. The rationale for these reverse views is obvious: A written response can be seen as evidence that may either get you into or out of legal trouble. An oral response, however, might get an employer into trouble, but no oral response is ever likely to get an employer out of legal trouble. The legal standard invariably encountered is that if a response cannot be verified by an official record—ordinarily an individual's personnel file—the response is inappropriate.

It remains a practice in some organizations that former supervisors are allowed to respond to reference inquiries. This is a hazardous practice. A former supervisor is a likely source of opinions, subjective assessments, and personality judgments, none of which are legally defensible if trouble arises. Reference requests should be handled centrally by the human resource department. As keeper of the official record—the personnel file—human resources is in a position to respond directly from the record and avoid all nonverifiable information. Repeat: Nothing that cannot be verified in a properly constituted official record should be provided in response to a reference request.

Often a manager in one organization will attempt to bypass normal reference processes by directly contacting his or her counterpart in another organization, thinking that what passes between colleagues without being committed to writing cannot possibly cause trouble. The manager who is tempted to go this route should consider this possible scenario: You exchange information with your counterpart, an individual is not hired based on what you said, and a legal action ensues. You find yourself in federal court under direct questioning as to what information you provided. What are you going to say? What will your counterpart say? The choices are committing perjury or admitting wrongdoing. Clearly it is far better to avoid the manager-to-manager reference check altogether.

Insight regarding performance may sometimes be obtained by asking whether the former employee is eligible for rehire. However, this practice is falling out of favor. Some organizations make it a policy to never rehire a former employee regardless of performance or reason for leaving. Sometimes, however, a negative response to the rehire question by the former employer may indicate performance issues. In this instance, the negative response should be probed with a follow-up request to clarify the reason for ineligibility, but that request may or may not be fulfilled depending on the policies or comfort level guiding the respondent.[10,11]

Conclusion

Fire rhymes with hire. There is but one letter difference between the two words, but this one letter makes a world of difference to both employer and employee. Surely hiring and being hired are far more pleasant than firing or being fired (see Chapter 8). But hiring done wrong can lead to an inevitable need to fire. This chapter is really about how to avoid that unpleasant outcome.

We have all often heard the expression, "It takes one to know one." This can be construed as a way of describing gut feelings. Gut feelings have their place in judging situations and people, but gut feelings alone can lead to improper interviewing, reference checking, and hiring decisions. Gut feelings must be balanced with knowledge of the business and the law, and trusting but verifying. Yet the experienced interviewer knows that if all of the answers seem right and the applicant looks good overall but there remains that uneasy feeling that something is not quite right, it is time to listen to the gut and start digging deeper.

Questions for Review and Discussion

1. Why is it frequently recommended that all reference requests be answered from one central location?
2. Why is it allowable to hire on the basis of favoritism? Under what circumstances should this not be done?

3. How and when did the fundamental rules for employee recruitment and selection change dramatically and permanently?

4. Generally describe the fundamental difference between legal and illegal interview questions.

5. What is the principal risk of overloading an interview with broad, open-ended questions?

6. Why is it not recommended to simply conduct credit history checks and general background checks on all applicants?

7. In some legal actions it is said, in effect, that if it is not in the permanent record, it never happened. Why?

8. Describe the differences between a job and a position. Can these terms ever have the same precise meaning?

9. Why is it said that the ability to carry on a conversation is evidence of one's ability to function as either interviewer or interviewee?

10. It has often been suggested that an employer can secure a measure of protection from legal problems by making a good-faith effort to check references. Describe a good-faith effort and indicate what this must absolutely include.

References

1. Merriam-Webster. (n.d.). *Interview*. Available at: http://www.merriam-webster.com/thesaurus/interview. Accessed November 2, 2009.

2. Kahn, S. C., & Brown, B. B. (2009). *Legal guide to human resources* (Vol. 1, pp. 2–42). Eagan, MN: Thomson Reuters/West.

3. Bureau of Law and Business, Inc. (1985). *How to write job descriptions . . . the easy way*. Madison, CT: Bureau of Law and Business, Inc.

4. Kethley, B. R., & Terpstra, D. E. (2005). An analysis of litigation associated with the use of the application form in the selection process. *Public Personnel Management, 34*, 357–376.

5. Kahn, S. C., & Brown, B. B. (2009). *Legal guide to human resources* (Vol. 1, 2: 61–62). Eagan, MN: Thomson Reuters/West.

6. Griggs v. Duke Power Co., 410 U.S. 424 (1971).

7. Kahn, S. C., & Brown, B. B. (2009). *Legal guide to human resources* (Vol. 2, 9:18). Eagan, MN: Thomson Reuters/West.

8. Babcock, P. (2003, October). The high cost of careless hiring. *HR Magazine*. Available at: www.shrm.org/Publications/hrmagazine. Accessed May 27, 2010.

9. Smith, A. (2007, March 29). EEOC urges caution on unnecessary credit checks. *HR News*. Available at: www.shrm.org/hrnews. Accessed May 27, 2010.

10. *The hiring handbook* (2nd ed.). (1995). New York: Aspen Publishers, Inc.

11. Burke, M. E. (2005). Getting to know the candidate: Providing reference checks. Available at: www.shrm.org/hrnews. Accessed May 27, 2010.

Chapter 7

Sexual Harassment: The Most Prevalent Form of Sex Discrimination

Clifford M. Koen, Jr., JD, MS, BBA, *Associate Professor of Business Law, East Tennessee State University, Johnson City, Tennessee*

Michael S. Mitchell, JD, LLM, *Attorney at Law and Partner, Fisher & Phillips LLP, New Orleans, Louisiana*

Stephen M. Crow, BS, MS, PhD, *Professor of Management, University of New Orleans, New Orleans, Louisiana*

Chapter Objectives

- Introduce sexual harassment as set forth in legislation and establish working definitions of sexual harassment.
- Review in some detail the various recognized forms of sexual harassment and establish the differences between and among them.
- Present guidelines to follow for the prevention of sexual harassment.
- Describe the essential contents of an effective sexual harassment policy.
- Set forth procedures by which to report, investigate, resolve, and document allegations of sexual harassment.

Introduction

Have we not heard enough about the legal intricacies associated with sexual harassment in the workplace? After all, healthcare organizations have navigated this challenging terrain for more than 40 years. The fact is we have not heard enough about sexual harassment; the legal environment of sexual harassment is still evolving. And pity the healthcare managers who do not keep up with this dynamic issue and find themselves lacking.

Although not involving a healthcare organization, the following is a recent attention-getting sexual harassment legal action against Hyundai Motor Manufacturing in 2009. The automaker took a $5.8 million hit, most of it in punitive damages.

> A federal jury . . . returned a $5.79 million verdict against Hyundai Motor Manufacturing and a mid-level manager for sexual harassment, negligence and retaliation. The jury awarded double what the plaintiffs were asking for . . . they were upset at the negligence. The (harasser) began harassing the (complainant) soon after her employment began in 2006.[1]

Was this an anomaly? Does it no longer happen often? Have organizations become more savvy about how to eliminate sexual harassment in the workplace? Not exactly. Discrimination charges filed with the Equal Employment Opportunity Commission (EEOC) for all categories reached an all-time high in 2008 at 95,402 charges.[2] Sexual harassment charges reached a 6-year high in 2008, about a 10% increase over the previous year.[3]

Liability for sexual harassment is usually very fact specific, and no brief review (such as what is presented in this chapter) can cover every aspect of this complicated topic. While not intended as a substitute for legal advice, this paper outlines the basic law pertaining to sexual harassment and provides practical advice to help prevent, recognize, and resolve claims of harassment.

Evolution of the Law

Title VII of the Civil Rights Act of 1964 prohibits discrimination in the workplace in hiring, firing, promotion, discipline, training, and other workplace decisions on the basis of sex, race, color, religion, and national origin. It was not until 1986 that the United States Supreme Court first held that Title VII's prohibition of sex discrimination included sexual harassment. The Supreme Court identified two types of sexual harassment: quid pro quo ("this for that") and hostile working environment. Since then, the EEOC (as the federal agency charged with enforcing this law) and the lower courts have wrestled with: (1) defining what behavior will be considered sexual harassment; (2) identifying who can be liable for harassment and under what circumstances; and (3) determining the potential scope of liability.

Sexual Harassment: Basic Principles

What Is Considered as Sexual Harassment?

The EEOC guidelines define sexual harassment as unwelcome sexual advances, requests for sexual favors, and other verbal or physical conduct of a sexual nature, when:

- Submission to such conduct is made either implicitly or explicitly a term or condition of employment;
- Submission to, or rejection of, such conduct by an individual is used as the basis for employment decisions affecting such individual; or
- Such conduct has the purpose or effect of unreasonably interfering with the individual's work performance or creating an intimidating, hostile, or offensive working environment.

This definition reflects the Supreme Court's analysis and has been widely adopted by the lower courts.

It is possible for an individual to also complain about harassment directed at others. This would arise when an employee complains because favoritism is shown to another employee who granted sexual favors or who may even be involved in a consensual relationship with a manager or supervisor. Courts have been reluctant to recognize this type of claim on the theory that preferential treatment for a lover is more akin to nepotism than sexual harassment.

On the other hand, where preferential treatment of employees who grant sexual favors becomes so pervasive that coworkers might reasonably conclude that granting sexual favors is the only way to advance in the organization or remain employed, courts are more likely to be sympathetic to a claim of third-party harassment.

In 1998, the Supreme Court recognized that Title VII also prohibits same-sex sexual harassment. It is important to remember that neither the harasser nor the victim needs to be homosexual in order for same-sex harassment to exist. Although these claims are not as prevalent as traditional male–female harassment, they are becoming more common. In 2008, males filed 15.9% of the sexual harassment charges brought to the EEOC. Therefore, prudent employers will treat all harassment complaints seriously.

For the sake of simplicity, all examples used in this chapter presume a female victim and male harasser. The following discussion, however, applies equally to the reverse or to a same-sex situation.

Examples of Conduct That Could Constitute Sexual Harassment

Determining whether particular actions constitute sexual harassment can be extremely difficult. The EEOC regulations do not make clear whether it takes one, two, or five sexually offensive comments or actions to constitute harassment. The Supreme Court has stated that Title VII does not affect "genuine but innocuous differences in the ways men and women routinely interact with members of the same sex and of the opposite sex." In other words, there is a certain amount of horseplay or simply annoying behavior that people must accept without legal redress.

Because of that, courts will look at several factors to determine if actionable harassment has occurred, including (1) the frequency of the discriminatory conduct; (2) the severity; (3) whether the conduct is physically threatening or a mere offensive utterance; (4) whether the conduct unreasonably interferes with an employee's work performance; and (5) the conduct's effect on the employee's psychological well-being.

Unfortunately, the line between actionable harassment and merely boorish behavior is drawn on a case-by-case basis and is often left to a jury. It is clear that the range of actions that could constitute sexual harassment is enormous and leaving such a determination to a jury is risky and expensive. Some common examples of conduct that might be deemed harassment include the following.

Physical actions:

- Touching a person's body, hair, or clothing;
- Hugging, kissing, or patting another;
- Standing close to or brushing up against a person;
- Touching or rubbing oneself in a private area or with sexual overtones near another person; or
- Touching, leaning over, cornering, or pinching someone.

Verbal actions:

- Referring to another as a "girl," "doll," "babe," "hunk," or "honey";
- Whistling or making catcalls at another;
- Making comments about a person's body, clothes, looks, anatomy, or manner of walking;
- Turning work discussions into sexual topics;
- Telling sexual jokes or stories;
- Asking about sexual fantasies, preferences, or history;
- Repeatedly asking a person for a date who clearly is not interested;
- Making kissing sounds, howling, or smacking lips; or
- Telling lies or spreading rumors about a person's sex life.

Nonverbal actions:

- Looking a person up and down (elevator eyes);
- Staring at someone;
- Blocking a person's path;
- Making sexual gestures with one's tongue or hands or other body movements;
- Following a person around;
- Giving unwanted personal gifts;

- Displaying sexually suggestive visuals (calendars, pictures, comics, food displays);
- Making facial expressions such as winking, throwing kisses, or licking lips; or
- Requiring an employee to wear provocative clothing.

Whether any of these or other possibly sexually related actions constitutes sexual harassment depends not only on their severity and whether they were isolated or repeated, but also on whether or not they were welcomed by the recipient.

Was the Conduct Welcome?

To be actionable harassment, the sexual behavior must have been unwelcome. Thus, determining whether the perpetrator's actions were welcomed by the recipient becomes a critical issue in determining whether behavior has gone from mutually consensual behavior to actionable sexual harassment. The Supreme Court has made it clear that submission to a sexual advance does not prove that the advance itself was welcomed. The Court recognized that a subordinate may voluntarily participate in a sexual act that is actually unwelcome because of the supervisor's threat (explicit or implicit) of adverse employment consequences. The correct inquiry is whether the recipient's conduct indicated that the sexual advances were unwelcome, not whether participation was voluntary.

A related issue questions whose perspective is to be used to determine whether the behavior was offensive or unwelcome. Is the concept of unwelcomeness judged from the perspective of the victim, the alleged harasser, or some reasonable person in society? The Supreme Court has stated that conduct must be unwelcome from the perspective of both the particular victim and of a reasonable person in the victim's situation. This analysis protects employers from liability from behavior found offensive by extremely sensitive victims who may not necessarily represent society's norms.

In determining whether the behavior was welcome, it is appropriate to examine the recipient's activities both before and after the alleged sexual advance. Unwelcome behavior might be demonstrated by facts such as the following:

- The employee did not solicit or incite the sexual advance;
- The employee regarded the advance as undesirable or offensive;
- The employee grimaced, frowned, or otherwise exhibited disagreement or resistance to the advance;
- The employee turned away or pretended not to hear the sexual comments;
- The employee pulled away, backed up, or attempted to avoid the perpetrator's touch;
- The employee complained to coworkers about the conduct; or
- The employee immediately complained to management about the incident or complained within a reasonable period under the circumstances.

It is important to understand that even if the recipient of the advance has dressed provocatively or has engaged in sexual horseplay with some coworkers, these activities do not necessarily mean that she welcomed the particular sexual behavior from the alleged harasser. The proper inquiry focuses on the recipient's response to the specific sexual advance(s) at issue. However, the victim's dress and behavior with others is not totally irrelevant in determining welcomeness, and juries can be adept in recognizing frivolous claims asserted by victims who use raw language or dress in a sexually provocative manner.

The difficulty with the welcomeness analysis can lie in the shifting perceptions of the alleged victim. If an employee is complaining, it is very likely she has been offended. More importantly, however, an employee's perception of events can depend upon a variety of factors including her relationship with the company. An employee who is open to sexual jokes may, on a later date when under fire for performance issues, claim she was offended. She then may report allegations of harassment in an attempt to make it difficult for the employer to terminate her for the unrelated performance issues. Because of this reality, an employer should foster an atmosphere with a level of professionalism and respect that eliminates discussion of potentially harassing topics at all times.

Under What Circumstances Can an Employer Be Held Liable for Sexual Harassment?

Title VII applies to private employers that "affect commerce" and have 15 or more employees, including part-time employees, for 20 or more weeks per year. The phrase "affect commerce" is construed very broadly and will encompass nearly all employers. Title VII also applies to most public employers regardless of the number of employees.

Many states and localities have their own statutes and ordinances patterned after Title VII covering companies with even fewer employees and frequently containing more stringent rules and definitions of prohibited conduct. Employers should never disregard a complaint of sexual harassment (unless advised otherwise by legal counsel) on the basis that the company has too few employees to be covered by any law (local, state, or federal) or because there is no employer–employee relationship with the complainant.

Note that under some circumstances, the law imputes an employer–employee relationship where no such relationship would otherwise exist. For example, under the concept of joint employer liability, if you exercise significant control over a worker, you could find yourself a legal coemployer of the individual. This often occurs in temporary employee leasing situations. Further, even persons that are considered independent contractors could actually be your employees, depending on the amount of control you exert over their daily activities.

Acts of Managers and Supervisors

Quid Pro Quo Sexual Harassment

Examples of this are:

- A manager's implication that an applicant's or employee's submission to sexual demands will cause her to be hired, promoted, or benefited in some way.
- A supervisor's suggestion to an employee that rejecting a sexual advance will result in her being disciplined, terminated, or economically harmed.
- An employee is demoted or reassigned to a less desirable shift or station after declining a supervisor's advances even though the employee's pay does not change.

Under the Supreme Court's most recent analysis, an employer will be held strictly liable for a manager's quid pro quo sexual harassment where the victim has suffered some job detriment. Whether the employer had notice of the harassment or expressly forbade it is irrelevant. Managers will be considered agents of the employer by virtue of their authority to act on behalf of the employer. Therefore, knowledge of a manager's actions that affect a victim's terms and conditions of employment will automatically be imputed to the employer.

Note that there is no defense in this situation (other than arguing that the harassment did not occur), and the only question at issue will be the amount of damages. This rule is harsh and emphasizes the importance of carefully selecting, supervising, and training your managers and supervisors.

The fact that a threatened adverse employment action was not actually carried out does not necessarily eliminate the employee's claim of harassment. Where no tangible employment action was taken, the employee can still claim that the supervisor's conduct created a hostile environment.

Hostile Environment Sexual Harassment

By creating a hostile environment, managers and supervisors can expose an employer to liability, even without conditioning an adverse employment action on the granting of sexual favors. A hostile environment is a situation where sexual harassment is so severe or pervasive that it alters the conditions of the victim's employment by creating an abusive working environment. The types of physical, verbal, and nonverbal conduct described in the previous section might all contribute to the creation of a hostile environment.

It is extremely important that employers adopt and enforce a written no-harassment policy to protect themselves from such hostile environment claims. Recent Supreme Court rulings provide employers an affirmative defense to a hostile environment claim as long as no tangible employment action has been taken against the employee. This defense allows an employer to avoid liability for a hostile environment where:

- The employer exercised reasonable care to prevent and promptly correct any sexually harassing behavior; and
- The victim unreasonably failed either to take advantage of any preventive or corrective opportunities provided by the employer or to avoid harm otherwise.

To ensure receipt of adequate and immediate notice of any potentially harassing behavior, employers should adopt, disseminate, and consistently enforce a written no-harrasment policy. The law clearly favors employers who have such a policy. When the victim knows that your company has a policy prohibiting harassment, but unreasonably fails to report the harassment, Title VII will allow you to use this as a defense against liability.

Acts of Coworkers

Quid Pro Quo Sexual Harassment

Unlike managers or supervisors, coworkers generally do not have the authority to affect conditions of employment. They generally cannot grant promotions, discipline, or terminate other workers. For this reason, nearly all quid pro quo cases involve allegations against a manager or supervisor.

There have been cases, however, where victims have claimed that coworkers engaged in quid pro quo sexual harassment. These generally involve situations in which a coworker and supervisor are friends and the coworker suggests to the victim that she would receive better training opportunities, better assignments, and better evaluations if she granted him sexual favors.

If a supervisor takes adverse action against the victim based upon a coworker's suggestions or recommendations, with knowledge of the coworker's request for sexual favors, courts have held the employer liable for the supervisor's actions. Thus, employers should ensure that employees understand (through a no-harassment policy and training) that no one in the organization has the authority to require sexual favors for job benefits and that such requests will not be tolerated.

Hostile Environment Sexual Harassment

Coworkers can also expose the company to liability for the hostile working environments they create. The standards for establishing liability on the part of coworkers are slightly different than for establishing liability on the part of supervisors. Particularly, notice to the employer of the harassment, either constructive or actual, is a requirement.

Actual notice occurs when you learn, either through an employee complaint or from observation (through your supervisors), that harassment is occurring. Constructive notice occurs when the facts or circumstances are such that any reasonable person in your shoes would or should have known that harassment was occurring. Constructive notice situations often involve employees who are loud and obnoxious and use sexually explicit, vulgar, or profane language. Although some coworkers may characterize individuals like this as eccentric or colorful, many others are often truly offended by such behavior.

It is important to understand that managers and supervisors have a duty to stop or, at a minimum, to report situations they observe that involve potentially harassing behavior. A supervisor's knowledge of harassment will in almost every instance be imputed to the employer.

The proactive steps an employer takes, such as adopting policies and conducting training, help in this area too. Thus, if the employer has a no-harrasment policy that includes a clearly defined reporting procedure, liability will generally be imposed only if a supervisor failed to investigate and take appropriate corrective action following receipt of actual or constructive notice of the harassment.

Acts of Nonemployees

Quid Pro Quo Sexual Harassment

Such claims could arise in situations in which the employer acts jointly with a non-employee to affect an individual's job because the individual either acquiesced or rejected the nonemployee's sexual advances. Some examples are:

- A doctor, client, or healthcare provider suggests that a business relationship with the employer will suffer unless one of the company's employees will engage in sexual liaisons.
- A favored customer asks the employer to terminate an employee because she rejected the customer's sexual advances.
- A vendor suggests that the employer would receive a better bargain if one of the company's employees acquiesced to the vendor's sexual advances.

Employers should ensure that all employees understand that harassment in any form, initiated by any person, whether employed by you or not, will not be tolerated and must be reported so that you can take appropriate corrective action.

Hostile Environment Sexual Harassment

While quid pro quo actions are unlikely, nonemployees can expose a company to liability by creating hostile working environments for its employees. These claims are made more troublesome because the company naturally wants to please its customers and keep vendors happy. Moreover, employers often lack significant control over nonemployee conduct. Some examples are:

- A cafeteria worker is repeatedly subjected to jeers, catcalls, groping, or lewd comments by customers.
- A nurse is repeatedly fondled or flashed by a patient.

As with other types of hostile environment claims, an employer can be liable for sexual harassment by nonemployees if the employer becomes aware of the harassment (through actual or constructive notice; in legal terms, a supervisor knew or should have known), and the supervisor fails to take appropriate corrective action.

Potential Damages

The company can be sued by a victim of sexual harassment under federal law; both the company and the alleged harasser can be sued under most state laws. A summary of the claims that can be made and the potential liability for each follows.

Under Federal Law

Under Title VII, as amended by the Civil Rights Act of 1991, a victim who proves that sexual harassment occurred can obtain an award of:

- Up to $300,000 in combined compensatory and punitive damages, depending on the size of the company (there are efforts in Congress to increase this cap);
- Back pay (for lost earnings from the time of termination until the lawsuit);
- Front pay (for lost earnings into the future for some reasonable period of time);
- Attorneys' fees and costs; and
- Appropriate equitable relief (such as an injunction or reinstatement).

Under State Law

Many states have statutes prohibiting discrimination modeled after, or similar to, Title VII. Some of these laws, however, do not have caps on the amount of damages that can be awarded. Thus, a plaintiff has incentive to seek redress in state court where the damages award can be much higher.

Additionally, victims of sexual harassment may be able to sue under the following additional types of state law claims, which are intended to protect persons from injury, including emotional and physical harm.

- Breach of contract: An employee who has an employment contract may be able to recover for a termination that violates the terms of that contract.
- Battery: Conduct resulting in harmful or offensive touching of another; grabbing, brushing against, touching, and fondling are typical claims.
- Assault: Conduct resulting in the imminent apprehension of a harmful or offensive contact; either verbal or physical harassment may constitute an assault.
- Intentional infliction of emotional distress: Behavior that is so shocking in character, or so extreme in degree, that a person of normal sensibilities would consider the action outrageous. Either verbal or physical harassment may constitute intentional infliction of emotional distress.

- Defamation: False statements about an individual that tend to damage reputation.
- Negligent hiring and retention: An employer's failure to fulfill a duty of reasonable care owed to employees or third parties, either by failing to investigate an applicant's background or by failing to take appropriate corrective steps when an employee has demonstrated a propensity for misconduct.
- Invasion of privacy: Conduct by which one person intrudes upon another's physical solitude or unnecessarily passes private information (whether true or false) about an individual to others.
- False imprisonment: Conduct in which one person confines another within the boundaries fixed by the first person, such as blocking someone's path, holding someone in a fixed place, or locking someone in a room.
- Loss of consortium: Claims by the victim's spouse that the spouse has been denied sexual relations by the victim as a result of the harassment.

It should be noted that the foregoing areas of the law may vary substantially from state to state. Also, for most of these types of claims, many states do not limit the type or amount of damages that may be awarded. This means that both compensatory damages and punitive damages may be awarded in any amount determined by the jury.

Claims by the Alleged Harasser

Although many males accused of harassment believe they should have a claim against the woman lodging the complaint or against the company that takes some form of disciplinary action against them, most courts do not agree. Alleged harassers have often tried to sue for defamation, wrongful discharge, and negligent investigation or discipline. With certain rare exceptions usually involving a totally frivolous complaint or a sham investigation, courts generally refuse to recognize such claims. The reasoning is that the law encourages the resolution of sexual harassment or discrimination complaints and will not punish the complainant or the employer for taking what was reasonably believed under the circumstances to be appropriate action.

Claims by Those Who Assist or Support the Rights of the Victim

Coworkers who support a victim in a claim of sexual harassment are also protected by the antiretaliation provisions of Title VII (and related laws). This is true whether the assisting employee gives the company a statement, gives the EEOC a statement, is interviewed on the employer's premises by the EEOC, or testifies at an agency hearing or in court. Thus, employers should act with care when imposing discipline or terminating employees following their involvement in a sexual harassment matter, and ensure that the discipline is warranted and proper under company policy and practice.

Guidelines for Preventive Action

Developing a No-Harassment Policy

There are several proactive measures employers can and should implement to help prevent sexual harassment from occurring and to reduce exposure when it does occur. Probably the most important measure is the adoption, communication, and consistent enforcement of a written policy prohibiting all forms of harassment. This policy should include the following.

Define Harassment. Some employers choose to use the EEOC definition of harassment, whereas others use plainer language and include examples of various kinds of harassment. Whichever approach you utilize, it is usually wise to include a prohibition of all types of harassment based on other criteria (e.g., religion, age, race, disability).

Prohibit Any Level of Harassment. The policy should communicate a zero tolerance stance. Many employers have found it beneficial to prohibit all sexual advances, not just those that are unwelcome.

State That Supervisors Do Not Have the Authority to Harass Employees. To avoid any possibility that employees may believe that a manager's actions are either impliedly approved or known by the company, the policy should specifically state that supervisors and managers do not have the authority to harass employees.

Outline Responsibilities. The policy should advise that all employees are obligated to report any harassment they observe, have heard about, or believe may be occurring.

Provide That Violators Will Be Disciplined Appropriately. The policy should state that disciplinary action will be taken up to and including discharge for conduct involving prohibited harassment. The appropriate level of discipline will generally depend on the severity of the harassment. If the harassment is a one-time relatively innocuous occurrence, verbal counseling (documented) or a written warning may be sufficient. If investigation reveals a pattern of similar harassing behavior or the conduct is aggravated, more severe discipline such as probation or even termination may be appropriate. In any harassment investigation, it is usually wise to seek legal advice.

Encourage Complaints. The policy should require all individuals who believe that they have been the victims of harassment, or who have observed or heard about harassment, to report it. In fact, somewhere in the policy, it should include the following in capital letters and in bold type: **DO NOT ASSUME THAT MANAGEMENT KNOWS ABOUT ANY PARTICULAR SITUATION. REPORT ALL INCIDENTS OF HARASSMENT.**

Assure That the Complaint Will Be Kept as Confidential as Possible. Never promise that the complaint or investigation will be kept strictly confidential. This is unrealistic and usually not possible. Rather, if the subject comes up, employers should advise that the complaint will be handled in a discreet manner and information will be kept on a need-to-know basis.

Provide Several Avenues of Complaint. One of the lessons of sexual harassment jurisprudence over the last several years comes from a common scenario present in many cases. Sexual harassment victims will report the conduct to someone in a supervisory role to whom they feel comfortable speaking. Many times, these complaints are accompanied by requests that the supervisors do nothing. This potential issue can be solved by training supervisors in identifying and properly responding to harassment issues. Once something is reported, action must be taken to at least investigate further.

The breadth of many employers' reporting procedures, telling employees to complain to any supervisor leads courts to conclude this was a proper report and put the employer on actual notice of the claim. Yet often, supervisory personnel do not respond properly claiming they did not think the conversation was a formal complaint.

Courts have also criticized policies that tell employees that they are obligated to report harassment up the ladder if nothing happens. For this reason, it is important to direct complaints to a place where you are confident that they will receive an appropriate response. Larger companies often provide toll-free numbers for this purpose. Smaller employers often direct these complaints to specifically named individuals in the human resources department. Whoever is listed as someone with authority to receive complaints of sexual harassment must be trained on how to properly respond. Given the sensitive nature of some sexual harassment, to help the victim feel at ease, it may be helpful to have at least one female and one male trained to receive complaints.

It is also important to provide an alternate means of complaint (such as directly to top management) if the employee is uncomfortable reporting to one of the specifically designated persons for some reason. This prevents a victim from asserting that the complaint reporting procedure could not be followed because she would have had to report the harassment to the alleged harasser.

Assure No Retaliation. Specifically assure that employees who, in good faith, report what they believe to be harassment, or who cooperate in any investigation, will not suffer retaliation. The policy should also state that any employee who believes he or she has been the victim of retaliation for reporting harassment should immediately report the retaliatory acts.

Require Employees to Acknowledge Receipt of the Policy and Agree to Abide by Its Terms. Requiring new hires to read and acknowledge receipt of all of the organization's rules and policies during their initial orientation is a good idea. You should have separate acknowledgment forms for supervisors and nonsupervisory employees. In the supervisor's acknowledgment, you may wish to add wording advising the supervisor that he or she might be held personally liable for engaging in sexual harassment.

Communicating the Policy

Once it is adopted, you should ensure that your harassment policy is communicated to employees in several ways. The policy should be posted on company bulletin boards, by time clocks, in lunch rooms, or in other areas where employees regularly congregate. During initial employee orientation, a manager should cover the policy in detail and encourage questions from new hires to ensure their understanding and acceptance of the policy. Managers should verbally communicate the policy at periodic supervisor and employee meetings, stressing each individual's responsibility for not engaging in prohibited behavior and reporting inappropriate behavior. Acknowledgment forms confirming receipt of the policy and agreement to report harassment or retaliation should be obtained from each employee and placed in employee personnel files.

Simply having a harassment policy is rarely going to be sufficient to establish that an employer took reasonable care to prevent sexually harassing behavior. In this area, the old adage "actions speak louder than words" is particularly true. If you are faced with a sexual harassment claim, your response to the claim will be critical to your defense. Supervisors who are not trained will not respond appropriately and their inadequate responses can often be more damaging than the conduct that gave rise to the complaint.

Supervisor training should be conducted on at least an annual basis. It need not be overly technical, but it should emphasize the priority the company places on preventing sexually harassing behavior. It should include training on the same elements that are included in a sexual harassment policy. Additionally, training should dispel common misperceptions about sexual harassment such as the need for an employee to make a formal complaint or the belief that a supervisor should acquiesce in an employee's request to do nothing. Finally, supervisors should be made aware that the company obligates them to report sexual harassment and the failure to do so could lead to disciplinary action against them.

Use of Love Contracts

An option used by employers in recent years to reduce the likelihood of sexual harassment suits is the love contract. Such contracts may be useful for top-level executives, but generally are not advisable for the average supervisor. Love contracts typically restate the consensual nature of the relationship, acknowledge existence of the employer's antiharassment policy, and state the policy that will be used if a problem arises. The subordinate agrees to release the employer from all claims that may arise from the relationship. An employer may want the parties to agree to resolve any work-related disputes using arbitration rather than resorting to the courts. Depending on the circumstances, love contracts may not be enforceable under the laws of some states. However, they may offer an employer some reasonable measure of protection.

Investigating Complaints

Generally, after sexual harassment has occurred, an employer's best defense to avoid liability is to take immediate and appropriate corrective action. A major issue with which an employer must contend is determining precisely what may be appropriate under the circumstances. To resolve this issue, the employer must conduct a proper and thorough investigation. Inaction is not an option.

There are four basic steps to handling a sexual harassment complaint: (1) taking the complaint; (2) interviewing the alleged offender; (3) investigating the complaint, including interviewing witnesses; (4) then taking appropriate action. Guide your investigation by ensuring that the following steps are followed and documented. Maintain all documentation in separate, confidential personnel files. Ensure that all interviews are conducted in private areas.

Taking the Complaint

- Assure the complainant that sexual harassment complaints are taken seriously by the employer.
- Listen carefully to the complainant's story. Put aside your personal biases and emotional responses and allow the person to speak candidly. Tactful and sympathetic demeanors are important, but express no opinion, make no assumptions, and make no commitment, other than to investigate the complaint.
- Consider having a witness in the room with you to take notes of the conversation. If the complainant is male, have a male witness. If the complainant is female, have a female witness. This will help make the employee more comfortable in discussing intimate or sexual matters.
- Be an active listener, asking open-ended questions, acknowledging the complainant's statements, and paraphrasing to ensure understanding.
- Get specific facts of the incident(s), including:
  - What the behavior was;
  - Where it occurred;
  - What effect the incident had on the victim;
  - Who was involved;
  - Any documentation or other physical evidence of the incident;

- When it happened (date and time);
- Whether there were witnesses (and who);
- Whether it has occurred before (if yes, when, over what period of time);
- Whether the complaining employee has told anyone else (if yes, who); and
- Did the complaining employee say anything to the alleged harasser to indicate that the behavior was unwelcome, uninvited, or offensive?

- Assess degree of welcomeness, if any, by determining what the complainant's response was to the harassment.
  - Did the complainant say anything to the alleged harasser to indicate that the behavior was unwelcome, uninvited, or offensive?
  - What was the complainant's physical response (i.e., did he or she turn away, laugh, smile)?
  - If the complainant said or indicated that the behavior was unwelcome, ask about the alleged harasser's response.

- Determine whether the complainant kept notes, and if so, ask to make a copy of them. If not, get as many details as possible and consider having the complainant sign pertinent notes from the interview. If the complainant has notes, find out when he or she began making the notes, whether the notes were kept contemporaneously with the event, how many pages exist, what type of book it is in (e.g., spiral bound, loose-leaf notebook), what color the outside of the book is, why he or she is keeping it, and whether he or she has written down every event of harassment. The purpose of obtaining minute details about such notes is to ensure that the complainant does not create an after-the-fact record of the alleged events that may be elaborated.

- Ask the employee if he or she thinks there are other individuals you should be interviewing, or if there is anything else that he or she believes you should know to more thoroughly investigate the matter.

- Determine credibility and demeanor of the complainant; note relevant comments and behavior.

- Ask how the complainant would like to see the situation resolved (i.e., what action the company should take to resolve the problem), but make no commitments on action to be taken.

- Assure the complainant that you consider the complaint a serious matter and that appropriate action will be taken as quickly and confidentially as possible.

- If the employee requests to have an attorney in the room to report the event, you should seek your own legal advice. Generally, it is not advisable to discuss this situation with an employee's lawyer; rather, you should discuss the guidelines and parameters of the interview with your own employment counsel.

- Offer no opinions; do not take sides.

- Ask the complainant to not discuss the investigation with any of the witnesses he or she has identified until you have spoken with them. This will help to keep the investigation as objective as possible.
- Tell the employee that you will inform him or her of the results of the investigation.

Interviewing the Alleged Harasser

- Remember that the accused has a right to hear and respond to the allegations, in detail.
- Conduct the interview in the same straightforward, unbiased manner as your interview with the complainant.
- Consider having a witness in the room with you to take notes of the conversation. Again, if the alleged harasser is male, have a male witness. If the alleged harasser is female, have a female witness. This may help make the alleged harasser more comfortable in discussing intimate or sexual matters.
- Be serious and to the point. Begin with something like, "The purpose of this meeting is to talk about an allegation of sexual harassment, which is a very serious matter." You do not want excessive small talk to signal that you do not consider this a serious matter.
- Do not initially identify the complainant.
- Get the names of witnesses.
- Determine credibility and demeanor.
- Focus on the alleged harasser's actual behavior rather than intent. Ask the accused to respond to each allegation separately and obtain the same type of information that you obtained from the complaining employee.
- Explain that no decisions have been made concerning the truthfulness of the complainant; remain unbiased.
- Find out whether the alleged harasser and the complainant socialize together (alone or in a group). If so, obtain details of the situations in which they have socialized.
- If the accused harasser admits to unlawful behavior, state that the behavior must stop immediately, and consider what will be appropriate disciplinary action.
- If the accused denies the behavior, explain that you now have two sides of the story and that you will be investigating further before making any determination. Caution the alleged harasser to not speak with coworkers regarding the allegation because any attempt to influence others could be construed negatively. Before disciplining anyone for discussing the complaint or investigation, however, you should consult labor counsel to ensure that any such discipline

will not violate the protected concerted activity provisions of the National Labor Relations Act.

- Advise the alleged harasser that the complaint and investigation will be kept as confidential as possible.
- Caution the alleged harasser strongly that the employer will not tolerate any acts of reprisal against the complaining employee or witnesses, if any.
- Consider having the accused sign a statement of or notes from the interview.

Interviewing Witnesses

- Do not initially identify the complainant. If possible, elicit the identity of the victim and the accused from the witness.
- Explain the serious nature of the situation.
- Ask what specifically did he or she see or hear and where it was witnessed (e.g., at work, away from work).
- Focus on first-hand observations, not assumptions. Note first-hand vs. second-hand knowledge.
- Determine credibility and assess demeanor.
- Find out if the witness is aware of any other potential sexual harassment involving others.
- Explain that the investigation is confidential and that discussing the matter may result in disciplinary action.
- Phrase questions in a way to avoid revealing any unnecessary information. Ask open-ended questions to determine what the witness knows, rather than obtaining yes or no confirmation of events you recite.
- Consider having the witness sign a statement of or notes from the interview.

Developing Information

- Monitor the workplace to ensure that the harassment (if any) stops and that no retaliation occurs. You may need to separate the two persons temporarily by reassigning one or the other until the matter is resolved. You should obtain legal advice in determining who to transfer to avoid retaliation claims for your actions.
- Try to speak with all of the witnesses and the parties' supervisor(s) as soon as possible (within the same day, if possible). Be as discreet as possible. Only interview witnesses who may have relevant information.
- If there are no witnesses, consider speaking with one or two trusted, long-term employees who may be able to provide insight into the behavior of both parties.

- As mentioned previously, before imposing any discipline for talking about the investigation, consult labor counsel to ensure that you do not violate the protected concerted activity provisions of the National Labor Relations Act.
- Do not limit the investigation to current employees. Interview former employees, friends, and relatives of both parties, if appropriate.
- Review and consider the personnel and supervisory files of both parties.
- Resist the temptation to accept or reject one side or the other until a full investigation is completed.

The importance of a proper investigation cannot be overstated. If facts are ascertained through a reasonable, good faith investigation, the employer will be better prepared to defend against claims of sexual harassment or claims brought by the alleged harasser for wrongful termination or defamation.

Taking Appropriate Action

If you conclude that harassment has occurred, you are legally obligated to take appropriate disciplinary action. Appropriate discipline may range from verbal counseling to immediate termination, depending on the severity of the circumstances, the parties' past records, and their positions within the organization.

If the complainant alleges employee harassment by a supervisor, you should:

- Ensure that whatever action taken is equitable, consistent with the employer's past practice, and appropriate under the law.
- Be prepared to explain fully the results of your investigation and the action that will be taken. If applicable, explain to the alleged harasser the right to appeal the decision to a higher level.
- Always communicate the results to the complainant with a reminder that she will not be retaliated against for bringing the complaint.
- Instruct the complainant to report any recurring or continuing harassment immediately.
- Monitor the workplace to ensure that the harassment has stopped and that no retaliation is occurring. Mark your calendar to check with the complainant regarding these issues at regular intervals for the following few weeks.
- Document carefully every step of the investigation and any subsequent action.

What constitutes appropriate corrective action for nonemployee harassment varies considerably depending on the circumstances, including the amount of control that you have over the nonemployee and the legal relationship between you and the nonemployee. You need to do whatever is reasonable under the circumstances to try to stop the harassment from occurring and clearly indicate to others that such conduct will not be tolerated. To reduce the risk of a defamation claim by the nonemployee, care should be taken to conduct a reasonable investigation before reporting the incident to the nonemployee's supervisor.

Reasonable corrective action may include the following:

- When the alleged harasser is a specific known individual (i.e., guest, patient, vendor), communicate directly with the individual to advise of your concern and request that the harassment stop. If the harassment continues, you may need to consider terminating your relationship with the nonemployee.
- When your employees complain that patients, vendors, or other third parties in general try to grope them or regularly make sexually suggestive remarks, you may need to evaluate your dress policies, post a no-harassment notice in a conspicuous place, and train your managers to police the environment.
- When the alleged harassers may be homeowners, patients, or business persons on your employee's route, you might consider allowing the employee to change the route, or assign those locations to other employees. If your employee's customers or patients change frequently (as in house calls for healthcare providers), you may need to consider including a no-harassment policy or notice in your customer or patient newsletter or correspondence.

Regardless of the type of situation, you must do whatever is reasonable under the circumstances to address and try to stop the harassment.

Taking Action Even if the Investigation Is Inconclusive

Even if the investigation is inconclusive (i.e., you have believable allegations sincerely brought, but no witnesses, and the alleged harasser credibly denies all allegations), you should still take proactive measures to ensure that employees understand their responsibilities and that the company takes such matters seriously. Consider the following steps:

- Write a memorandum for each employee's file documenting the investigation. Make a record of the relevant facts, including factors that are considered to have raised suspicion.
- Write separate memoranda to the complaining party and the alleged harasser, placing copies in your confidential investigation file. The memoranda should include:
  - The fact that the investigation was inconclusive, but will remain open in case other information surfaces that will assist the company in making a final determination;
  - A reminder of the company's no-harassment policy, attaching another copy for their reference;
  - An expectation that no other harassment complaints against the alleged harasser will surface in the future. Also include an assurance that if any complaint is made, the company will take immediate appropriate action; and
  - A reminder that retaliation will not be tolerated.

- Meet with each individual separately and communicate the results of the investigation, the action that will be taken, and the content of the memoranda discussed previously.

Questions for Review and Discussion

1. When can apparently consensual sexual activity actually involve unwanted behavior that constitutes sexual harassment?
2. What is the legal position of the organization if top management knows nothing about sexual harassment that may be occurring among workers and first-line managers?
3. What is the importance of having thorough documentation of every step from reporting sexual harassment to final resolution of a complaint?
4. As a manager, what should you do if an employee tells you of sexual harassment but also tells you to say nothing to anyone about it?
5. When can asking a coworker for a date be considered sexual harassment?
6. How is sexual harassment covered under the conditions of Title VII of the Civil Rights Act of 1964?
7. What danger, if any, is inherent in a long-term fully consensual affair between employees?
8. What recourse is available to an employee whose alleged harasser is also that person's immediate supervisor?
9. How can a supposedly hostile environment exist if no one says or does anything directly harassing?
10. What are some key considerations that can turn supposedly innocent behavior into actionable sexual harassment?

References

1. Gordon, R. K. (2009, May 5). Jury rules against Hyundai. *The Birmingham News*. Available at: http://www.al.com/business/birminghamnews/news.ssf?/base/business/1241511326232950.xml&coll=2. Accessed December 29, 2009.
2. US Equal Employment Opportunity Commission. (n.d.). *Sexual harassment charges, EEOC & FEPAs combined: FY 1997–FY 2009*. Available at: http://www.eeoc.gov/eeoc/statistics/enforcement/sexual_harassment.cfm. Accessed December 29, 2009.
3. US Equal Employment Opportunity Commission. (n.d.). *Charge statistics, FY 1997 through FY 2009*. Available at: www.eeoc.gov//eeoc/statistics/enforcement/charges.cfm. Accessed December 29, 2009.

Chapter 8

Discipline and Discharge: "You're Fired!" Is Not That Easy

Bianca Perez, MS, *Doctoral Candidate, Public Affairs Program, University of Central Florida, Orlando, Florida*

Aaron Liberman, PhD, *Professor, Department of Health Management and Informatics, University of Central Florida, Orlando, Florida*

Chapter Objectives

- Introduce the foundations of progressive discipline.
- Describe applications of progressive discipline and the circumstances under which certain forms of it apply.
- Review the steps of the progressive disciplinary process.
- Enumerate guidelines for the structure and operation of progressive discipline systems and identify organizational obstacles to its use.
- Review the legal ramifications of progressive discipline and provide guidelines for the manager's legal application of disciplinary action.
- Identify alternate forms of progressive discipline and their applications.
- Develop understanding of the all-important role of accurate, complete, and objective documentation in applying disciplinary action.

Introduction

Before discussing employee discipline, two concepts must be introduced. The first is performance management, a systematic approach to identifying employees' strengths and weaknesses in addressing an organization's goals, as well as the variables that may compromise the realization of those aspirations.[1]

The second concept to consider is counterproductive workplace behavior; in other words, infractions of rules or policies and, in general, negative actions committed by an employee that may disrupt normal activities or ultimately harm the organization.[2] It is the deliberate nature of harmful behaviors that distinguishes these behaviors from performance problems resulting from a lack of knowledge, skill, or ability. Problems of performance are generally addressed via teaching, coaching, and counseling; it is primarily violations of rules or policies that are addressed through disciplinary processes.

Taking the foregoing concepts into consideration, the disciplinary process may thus be described as a critical activity undertaken to eliminate negative and egregious behaviors to ensure a more productive and capable workforce.

Many managers are understandably apprehensive about the disciplinary process, but the reluctance to deal with inappropriate behavior only exacerbates the problem. Disciplinary problems are often poorly addressed for two reasons. Managers sometimes fail to address problem behavior promptly and consistently, ultimately compromising productivity and employee morale.[3] At other times, errant behavior may cause a manager to react impulsively by attempting to prematurely terminate the employment relationship. However, in truly serious circumstances involving blatantly dishonest or criminal acts resulting in significant damage to property or harm to employees or others, the organization is justified in immediately severing the employment relationship to minimize harm and perhaps to minimize the organization's liability for illegal conduct. Less severe instances of behavior may be dealt with progressively. Thus, if an errant employee is both willing and able to correct the offending conduct, then working *through* the problem can be worthwhile. Although a question of judgment arises as to whether an employee is truly ready and willing to commit to enduring change, the negative repercussions of termination— including increased turnover cost, loss of training investment, and reduction in employee morale—are reminders that employee retention is far more desirable than termination.

Progressive Discipline

Benefits

Progressive discipline provides for a series of responses to inappropriate employee behavior ranging from mild to severe that can eventually result in termination of employment. Progressive discipline is consistent with B. F. Skinner's view that people, like other creatures, are less likely to repeat behaviors that are associated with negative outcomes.[4] Therefore, progressive discipline is commonly associated with behavior modification techniques.

Progressive discipline may also reduce legal risks and increase the defensibility of the organization's termination procedures. One of the difficult challenges encountered in terminating employees is the need to deal with the issues of *just cause* and *due process*.[5] Specifically in the event of a wrongful discharge lawsuit, the employer must prove that an aggrieved employee was made aware of the behavioral deficiency *and* was given sufficient opportunity to correct the offending behavior. Except for addressing infractions deserving immediate discharge, the primary purpose for using progressive discipline is *correction of behavior*. There are, however, peripheral benefits such as improved communication, improved morale, and more favorable retention rates.

Ethical Considerations

There are occasionally some erroneous assumptions that can cause the disciplinary process to go awry. First, "behavior modification" has historically been criticized on the grounds that it is a mind-controlling process that prevents individuals from exercising free will; some authorities claim that *systematically* modifying behavior is unethical. In contrast, proponents of behavior modification assert that this technique is actually intended to foster independence and self-control.

The second assumption that needs to be challenged is that discipline is equivalent to punishment. The word *punishment*, of course, carries a generally negative connotation for most people, while *correction*, although negative to some, comes across more positively than punishment. No matter the extent to which the corrective intent of discipline is stressed, however, there will be a visible element of punishment every time an employee is discharged for a single, serious infraction. This can be obliquely construed as correction only in the sense that a problem is "corrected" by removing its source.

Progressive Discipline and the Law: A Guide for the Manager[6]
Nonunion Setting

Generally, to uphold a disciplinary action, including discharge, courts typically look for: (1) consistency; (2) clear and convincing documentation of unacceptable performance or behavior; as well as proof that (3) the employee was aware of the employer's expectation; (4) the employee was informed about the unacceptable performance or behavior; and (5) the employee was given reasonable opportunity to improve to meet the employer's expectations.

Unionized Setting

The key issue concerned with disciplinary action in a unionized setting is usually whether the discipline in question was for just cause. The concern over just cause refers to language typically found in the collective bargaining agreement.

Generally, to determine whether just cause exists in a disciplinary action, three elements must be considered: (1) the employee must be provided with due process, that is, the process used must be fair in form and application; (2) there must be sufficient evidence of the unacceptable performance or behavior; and (3) action chosen by the employer must be appropriate under the circumstances, that is, the severity of the action must be consistent with the severity of the infraction.

A system that is fair and is uniformly and fairly applied to all employees will be less likely to be attacked by disgruntled employees and will likely result in a legally valid disciplinary action if challenged in court.

Determining Just Cause

What constitutes just cause is usually defined on a case-by-case basis. However, an often-cited and well-established measure of this concept is commonly known as the Seven Tests of Just Cause. The following factors are considered:

1. Notice. Did the employer give the employee reasonable warning of the possible or probable consequences of the employee's conduct?
2. Reasonable rule. Was the employer's rule or managerial order reasonably related to (a) the orderly, efficient, and safe operation of the business, and (b) the performance that the employer might reasonably expect from the employee?
3. Investigation. Did the employer, before taking disciplinary action, make an effort to determine whether the employee actually violated or disobeyed a rule or order of management?
4. Fair investigation. Was the employer's investigation conducted fairly and objectively?
5. Proof. In the investigation, did the employer obtain substantial evidence that the employee was guilty as charged?
6. Equal treatment. Has the employer applied its rules, orders, and penalties evenhandedly and without discrimination?
7. Appropriate penalty. Was the degree of discipline administered by the employer reasonably related to (a) the seriousness of the employee's proven offense and (b) the record of the employee's service with the employer?

The foregoing seven issues can be considered in analyzing the circumstances in terms of fairness and due process. A "no" answer to one or more of these questions means that just cause was either not satisfied or at least was seriously weakened in that some arbitrary, capricious, or discriminatory element was present. And even though these factors originally arose in an arbitration (union) setting, they are fully as applicable in nonunion settings as well. The 25 questions appearing in Exhibit 8-1 expand upon the seven issues and include some of the most important questions that every manager should ask before proceeding with a significant disciplinary action.

Exhibit 8-1

Discipline and Termination Checklist

1. Do I have all the facts, and has a thorough investigation been conducted to verify those facts?

2. Is the proposed disciplinary action for this employee consistent with the treatment others have received for the same offense and/or in the same department or other department?

3. What is the employee's past disciplinary record?

4. What is the employee's service record?

5. Is the rule that has been violated a reasonable one?

6. Has the rule been applied in a reasonable way in this case?

7. Did the employee know the rule? If not, is it reasonable to think the employee should have known the rule?

8. Has the employee been given fair warning (preferably in writing) concerning the seriousness of his or her conduct? (This would not apply for serious misconduct, such as fighting on the job or sabotage, where there is irrefutable proof.)

9. Was there a record made of such past warning, and is it on file? Who gave the warning? When?

10. Have similar past violations resulted in little more than verbal reprimands or even been overlooked?

11. Does my organization have a past record of strict enforcement for similar offenses? If not, have employees been warned of the intention to strictly enforce the rule?

12. Have I observed all rules and followed proper preliminary procedures including my employer's disciplinary policies and procedures?

13. Was there a personal problem that may have contributed to the employee's action?

14. Does the employee have a reasonable excuse?

15. Was the employee given a reasonable opportunity to improve?

16. Was the employee offered a reasonable amount of help and did the employee take advantage of that help?

17. Did the employee know what was expected of him or her?

18. Am I being fair, unbiased, and levelheaded, or am I reacting against the employee?

19. Can I prove the employee's guilt by direct, objective evidence, or am I relying only on circumstantial evidence or suspicion?

(continues)

20. What effect will the discharge (or failure to discharge) have on other employees and how will it affect morale?

21. Is the timing of the discharge correct (for example, to avoid the appearance of retaliation)?

22. Does the punishment fit the crime?

23. What possible alternative is there to discharge?

24. Are we dealing with a potential claim of employment discrimination or wrongful discharge? For example, could factors such as age, gender, race, religion, disability, or national origin be an issue?

25. Do I need assistance from my superior, the human resources department, or outside counsel?

Source: Adapted from Koen, C. M., Jr., & Mitchell, M. S. Supervisor's Checklist for Termination/Discipline, *SuperVision*, 27(1), January 2010, with permission of copyright holders C. M. Koen, Jr., and M. S. Mitchell.

Steps Involved in Progressive Discipline

The commonly employed progressive discipline model consists of four steps for addressing employee transgressions: oral warning, written warning, suspension, and termination. At every step, the manager needs to address the issue with the employee face-to-face. Second-hand discipline—writing up an infraction just to place in a file—has no place in the management of people. It is also of paramount importance to carefully document every step of the process, including the oral warning. One might ask why it is necessary to document a supposed oral warning; this is done to enable the manager (or human resources) to present evidence that this step of the process was utilized before additional steps were taken.

Oral Warning

This is typically where the progressive disciplinary process begins. The manager notifies the employee that a problem exists and offers counseling and training to help overcome the problem. In this step, the discrepancy between expected and actual behavior is delineated; cooperation is requested from the employee; the employee is asked to provide an explanation of the behavior; the employee's questions are answered; further consequences are outlined; and the time frame in which behavior is expected to change is spelled out. The resulting document—to be retained by the manager and not submitted for the individual's personnel file—should include the date and purpose of the meeting, the nature of the deficiency, the suggested means of eliminating the problem, and, ideally, the employee's signature.

Written Warning

If the offending behavior persists, or if the transgression is severe enough to *begin* with this step, a written warning is generated. This makes reference to the previous warning and specifies the next step in the disciplinary process. The written warning should include a description of the expected corrective action, a future date to evaluate the results, a statement offering assistance in overcoming the problem, and a statement identifying the resources that may be available to help the employee.

Suspension

If the errant behavior persists, or if misconduct is serious enough for the process to start at an advanced stage, the manager may opt to suspend an employee so as to send a stronger message. Suspension emphasizes the seriousness of the problem by causing the individual to experience temporary severance from employment. Suspension may occur with or without pay depending on the organization's policy. It is suggested, however, that the strongest message involves suspension *without* pay for a period not to exceed 1 workweek. Some employees, especially those who have no thought of spending an entire career with the present employer, are likely to regard suspension *with* pay as extra paid vacation. Sometimes, however, when an employee is suspended *pending an investigation*, the individual may be paid.

Termination

Termination occurs either when misconduct is severe—the organization's policy usually enumerates those infractions that call for immediate termination—or when the steps of the progressive process have been exhausted but the offending behavior continues. Termination should never come as a surprise to the employee; either the behavior is so serious that termination is the obvious recourse, or the employee has already received numerous warnings about the problem. In many instances it is advisable to hold the termination discussion in the presence of multiple parties for safety and security reasons and to provide one or more witnesses in case legal challenges arise.

In Implementing Progressive Disciplinary Systems

Progressive disciplinary systems must be implemented in a manner that enhances employee perceptions of fairness, accuracy, and effectiveness.

First, any progressive discipline process must be applied consistently. A manager who overlooks an instance of inappropriate behavior by one employee and later reprimands another for the same infraction is creating a breeding ground for discrimination complaints. This highlights the importance of managers' awareness of the federal laws that prohibit discrimination on any basis. Also, research has shown that managers who overlook one instance of inappropriate behavior are more likely to condone future instances of the same behavior.

Discipline should be promptly initiated so that the errant employee clearly sees the connection between misconduct and consequences. Delay dilutes the effectiveness of any disciplinary action.

Occasionally, however, immediate responses to infractions are not advisable. The onset of formal disciplinary action should be delayed if either employee or manager is obviously angry. An employee who is angry or extremely upset is not completely rational and is thus more difficult to deal with, and anger on the part of the manager can cloud judgment and skew objectivity. It should be accepted as a rule that a manager should never reprimand or discipline in anger.

An Alternative Form of Progressive Discipline

Behavioral Contracting

Behavioral contracting is a behavior modification technique whereby written agreements serve to clearly outline contingencies between behaviors and their consequences.[7] Behavioral contracting originated in the fields of psychology and social work as *contingency contracting* and was used to address a wide array of problems, such as eliminating addictive behaviors, generating patient compliance in health care, modifying classroom behaviors, and improving family relationships. Its potential for eliminating deviant work behaviors and for improving employee relations can be readily inferred.

Behavioral contracting in the workplace has been described as "*a direct, structured method for enforcing a required change of performance or attitude . . .* and *represents a natural sequence of steps in which the manager and employee . . . come to an agreement that change is necessary for an employment relationship to continue.*"[8] Given this definition, behavioral contracting in the workplace should primarily be used to address more serious types of infractions. Behavioral contracting stands in contrast to zero-tolerance policies in that an errant employee is given an opportunity to rectify inappropriate behavior before being terminated.

Compared with progressive discipline, however, behavioral contracting does not involve a series of responses of increasing severity. Behavioral contracting offers benefits similar to progressive discipline in that it eliminates inappropriate behavior, improves work performance, enhances job satisfaction, increases perceptions of fairness, and reduces the organization's susceptibility to legal actions. Furthermore, given the emphasis on creating a contract, behavioral contracting ensures that parties are aware of their obligations and the behavioral conditions that apply, and can ensure improvement of the relationship between the parties. Overall, given the serious nature of the behavior that triggered the onset of formal discipline, the employee is often grateful to have been given a chance to salvage the employment relationship.

There are seven significant steps in the behavioral contracting process.[8] The first step involves intervention by the manager to educate the employee: The unacceptable behaviors are unequivocally described and outlined, and it is made clear to the employee that continued employment is dependent upon behavioral change.

The second stage centers on the degree of the employee's acceptance of responsibility for the behavior. In this stage, the manager may observe a wide range of employee reaction. If sincere expressions of regret are noted, progress has been made. If denial or fakery arises, the antecedents of the behavior should be outlined so that the employee can realize his or her contribution to the situation.

In the third stage, the interaction becomes collaborative as employee and manager make a joint effort to identify the problems surrounding the behavior in the most factual manner possible. Perceptual differences often arise as the employee tries to attribute the root cause of the behavior to an external source. As the manager questions the validity of the excuses individually, most affected employees will eventually recognize the extent of their contribution to the problem.

In the fourth stage, the contract is crafted. The contract is not imposed on the employee; rather, it is jointly written. The contract should include several components: specific benchmarks for future behavior, the process by which behavior will be monitored, the information to be collected, and how progress will be assessed. Signatures of both parties are required to seal the contract.

The fifth stage is the observation period during which manager and employee periodically meet to assess behavioral developments. The manager's feedback should clarify what the employee has yet to accomplish and acknowledge any progress that is realized by the employee.

The sixth stage usually signifies resolution of the problem. This stage consists of a formal meeting in which the manager expresses satisfaction and commends the employee for accomplishing the goals set out in the contract. The manager may opt to tear up the contract and discard it, indicating that the matter is closed. But whether the contract is or is not discarded, the behavioral contracting process provides an indelible experience affecting the employee at a fundamental level.

Overall, behavioral contracting has proven to be effective for altering behavior; however, it also has its limits. Specifically, behavioral contracting may not necessarily have generalized effects across different settings or behaviors. Thus, managers should not expect that the entire gamut of inappropriate behaviors will be eliminated with a single execution of behavioral contracting. Although behavioral contracting signals the seriousness of behavioral infractions to employees, it may only effectively eliminate the specific behaviors outlined in the contract.

Precautions with Behavioral Contracting

Behavioral contracting, quite likely beyond the immediate capabilities of many first-line managers, is not without its hazards. Depending on the law of the state where this is utilized, forming such a contract could have legal implications; it could conceivably be deemed a legal and binding contract and create a greater problem than the manager is attempting to address. The behavioral contract unearths potential issues that make its use risky; for example, discarding the contract to indicate that the matter is closed may not be as simple as it sounds. The contract may be torn up, but the resulting legal problems may be just beginning.

Behavioral contracting is perhaps best considered for higher-level employees, such as certain technical or professional staff. Also, if the manager uses this approach with one employee, it must at least be considered for others, and if it is not so used, the reasons for choosing not to use it in any particular instance should be documented. The fact remains that *consistency* in how discipline is administered is always a key consideration because inconsistent application can result in claims of disparate treatment.

Outcomes of Disciplinary Incidents

Practical Outcomes

The benefits of a carefully designed progressive discipline system affect every level within an organization. At the department level, efficiency is increased and the amount of supervisory time consumed by people problems is decreased. At the individual level, employees who have experienced discipline are often mindful of having been given a second chance as well as an opportunity for growth. Progressive discipline can also improve communication between managers and employees and improve morale and retention by demonstrating fairness and consistency in dealing with performance issues. Also, disciplinary actions can have more far-reaching implications in that they allow organizations to communicate their work ethic to the public. Specifically, organizations that maintain high performance standards tend to retain and attract employees who share the same work ethic.

Making Examples

There are perhaps a few managers here and there who apparently believe—quite erroneously—that public disciplining (i.e., disciplining in the presence of others) has positive vicarious effects on coworkers. The effects of public disciplining, however, are usually limited to added embarrassment for the errant employee, resentment in those who witness the act, and general diminution of respect for the manager. It should be accepted as a given that discipline should always be carried out in private, strictly between manager and offending employee. One of the poorest employee relations moves a manager can make is to hold up an employee as an example for others.

Perceptions of Organizational Justice

The issue of organizational justice is crucial to understanding the consequences of formal disciplinary procedures. Employees' willingness to change depends considerably on whether they perceive that they have been treated fairly. Organizational justice has three components. There is interactional justice, which refers to perceived fairness of treatment as typified by a manager's good manners and respectful treatment of the employee. The second component is procedural justice, referring to employee perceptions of the relative fairness in the way policies are applied and decisions are carried out. Policies that are applied consistently and without bias increase employees' perceptions of fairness. The third component is distributive justice, which relates to the perceived fairness of the outcomes of a process; that is, that the perception of the severity of the manager's response is consistent with the severity of the infraction and that the disciplinary procedures apply equally to all employees.

Perceived Effects on the Psychological Contract

Rousseau defined the psychological contract as *"An individual's belief regarding the terms and conditions of a reciprocal exchange agreement between the focal party and another party. A psychological contract emerges when one party believes that a promise of future returns has been made, a contribution has been given and thus, an obligation has been created to provide future benefits."*[9]

Psychological contracts are separate from the employment contract and largely exist in the mind of an employee in the form of beliefs and expectations. Psychological contracts are based on reciprocal exchanges between employee and employer, and they exist even if neither party acknowledges their presence. Employees perceive that employment itself constitutes the promise and that their work performance constitutes the contribution.

The importance of psychological contracts is such that without promise of a future exchange, neither the employee nor the employer has an incentive to continue the work relationship. Although their inception cannot be pinpointed, psychological contracts are formed in every employment relationship because of the gaps that exist in all employment arrangements. Despite the elusive and hypothetical nature of psychological contracts, neither their existence nor their impact on employment relationships can be denied.

With respect to discipline, psychological contracts may create an expectation that employees are entitled to opportunities to rectify inappropriate behavior. If this assumption is correct, progressive discipline would be an effective way to ensure that an organization fulfills its implied promises. Because such disciplinary methods are progressive in nature and centered on learning, their fair and consistent use can increase employee perception of trust in the employment relationship. Although psychological contracts are merely implied agreements that have no legal standing, perceived violations can have repercussions for organizations including decreased job satisfaction, eroded trust, poor perceptions of procedural justice, and increased turnover rates. Psychological contracts cannot be eliminated and cannot be ignored.

Challenges Inherent in Disciplining Employees

Thus far, this chapter has suggested that although progressive discipline is an effective way to address inappropriate employee behavior, disciplining employees is a complex process and can be a paralyzing task for managers. There are several obstacles that need to be overcome to facilitate the employee discipline process.

Interpersonal Obstacles

Most managers find disciplining employees unpleasant, so they sometimes rationalize avoidance of the process. Common rationalizations are abundant: "Why should I be the only manager to discipline?" "Why devote the time and effort to a minor infraction?" "If I wait a while the problem may just go away." "What if the employee becomes angry with me?" No manager likes to intentionally be the bad guy. Managers often fear the way in which they will be perceived by an employee who must be disciplined, and they are sometimes afraid disciplining will harm their relationships with employees. However, if one accepts good relationships as based on mutual respect and fair dealing, then the disciplinary process should by no means be perceived as threatening such relationships.

When one cuts through all of the rationalizations and excuses, it all boils down to the necessity to exhibit sufficient courage to humanely do what is necessary, fair, and right regardless of potential employee reactions. In all disciplinary actions, and indeed in all instances in which deserved criticism is called for, the manager must act with courage and compassion—the courage to do what is necessary and the compassion to do it with kindness and consideration.

Organizational Obstacles

The greatest potential obstacle is lack of organizational support. Support for disciplining employees should sustain management efforts to properly practice employee discipline. Explicit support should be discernible through formal policies communicated both verbally and in writing and should be found throughout all levels of an organization's structure. Under conditions of positive support, a manager who properly carries out disciplinary action will not be questioned unnecessarily by superiors or, in the worst-case sense, be overruled by higher management.

Implicit in the foregoing paragraph is the absolute necessity for the full support of higher management for the proper application of disciplinary action. The manager who must discipline an employee must have the support of superiors as well as the support, guidance, and, often, assistance of the human resources department.

Another organizational obstacle often encountered is inadequate or nonexistent training of managers in dealing with problem employees. Training in the specifics of the organization's formal disciplinary process should be considered a must for every manager and especially for first-line managers, those who directly supervise the people who do the hands-on work. All employees, including managers, should be periodically reminded of the organization's standards of conduct and behavior.

Sometimes there are obstacles created by the organization's culture, that collection of shared beliefs, values, norms, and expectations that guide organizational behavior. The organizational culture can produce variations in the way employee discipline is carried out. For example, if an organization openly sanctions the use of disciplinary action in its policy manual but on a tacit level fails to apply discipline consistently or at all, it will inevitably send managers conflicting cues about how to proceed. This, in turn, produces inconsistencies in the way disciplinary action is carried out.

Motivations of managers represent another potential source of obstacles. Many managers who are knowledgeable of disciplinary processes and are thus capable of providing negative feedback are often unwilling to do so because they feel the organization does not value such efforts. Also, managers who, for a variety of reasons, remain uneasy about dispensing criticism undermine the system by disciplining too late, too little, or not at all.

Legal Issues

The recent three decades have seen a significant level of employee complaints alleging wrongful discharge. Amendments to legislation plus numerous court decisions have enabled aggrieved former employees to secure increasingly lucrative damage awards for having been discharged in bad faith. Overall, employment-related complaints have been increasing for a number of years, consistent with the increasingly commonplace litigiousness of American society in general. Indeed, one of the strongest forces at work in holding many managers back from giving serious disciplinary issues the full attention they deserve is the fear of being sued.

Many states have enacted the *employment-at-will* doctrine, which maintains that both the employee and the employer can terminate the employment relationship at any time and for any reason.[1] However, the judicial concept of a wrongful discharge has proven nebulous because it leaves room for employers to terminate employees for questionable reasons and has enabled terminated employees to retaliate against their former employers when, in fact, their behavior truly warranted discharge.

There are three main judicial exceptions to the employment-at-will doctrine. First is the *implied contract exception*, which states that any written or verbal understanding that creates an expectation of job security cannot be arbitrarily disregarded by an organization.[10] An implied contract can exist, for example, when an organization tells its employees via handbook or policy manual or perhaps even at employee orientation that discharges occur solely for just cause. Such statements have frequently been considered to represent implied contracts of employment.

The second judicial exception applies to every employment relationship and places even greater restrictions on the definition of at-will employment, the *covenant-of-good-faith exception*. The interpretation of this exception is somewhat unclear.

Some courts have ruled that employers always require just cause to terminate an employee, but others have declared an outright prohibition against termination motivated by malice. Both the implied contract and covenant-of-good-faith exceptions to the employment-at-will doctrine hold implications for managing problem employees because they remind organizations that discipline should always be dispensed with good intentions and should never be administered capriciously.

The third judicial exception is the *public policy exception*, recognized in both court cases and legislation, for terminations that violate the public policy of the state. Violations of public policy typically arise when the employee is terminated for refusing to violate a criminal statute on behalf of the employer or for engaging in activities such as reporting employer violations of statutes or reporting other employer wrongdoing (i.e., for whistle-blowing). This exception is recognized in more than 40 states and is usually associated with employer actions that are malicious or retaliatory.

Documentation: The Critical Defense

Picture the following scenario: A department manager visits the organization's human resources director with a litany of complaints about an employee. The employee, says the manager, is uncooperative and unreliable, is frequently absent without apparent cause, and exhibits conduct that, at times, approaches insubordination. This employee's work is only marginally acceptable at best, and, overall, this person has been a continuing source of problems. The manager has finally "had it," and passes a single sheet of paper—a discharge notice—to the human resources director. This employee "has got to go."

The director first asks whether any of the employee's infractions have been among the serious ones calling for immediate discharge, such as theft, fighting, or being under the influence of alcohol. The employee has not and has done nothing of an ultimately serious nature but rather, has piled up a lengthy string of minor-to-moderate infractions.

The director then asks for the manager's documentation. The manager indicates the single sheet—the discharge notice just presented. The manager admits to never having written up a single infraction, suggesting that "writing up every little problem is a royal pain," but reiterates that for the good of the organization and its patients, this employee must go. Now.

The director refuses to sanction discharge of this employee. There have been no earlier indications of trouble, no counseling memos, no documents describing oral warnings, no written warnings, no implemented suspensions, nothing until this single "final" document. There is even in the employee's file a brief, marginally satisfactory performance evaluation that cites no problems, but nowhere in the file is there any indication that this person has ever been warned about inappropriate behavior or given the opportunity to work toward correction. The organization has absolutely no means of legally supporting discharge; the manager must essentially start over with this employee, going back to square one and utilizing counseling and disciplinary processes when inappropriate behavior occurs.

As noted earlier in this chapter, the fundamental assumption that arises whenever appropriate documentation cannot be produced in support of a disciplinary action is "If it is not documented, it never happened." This assumption can prevail in court and ensure a loss for the organization.

As disciplinary processes must be applied when behavior is deserving of such, each step must be properly documented as it occurs. If no documentation exists concerning the behavior of a misbehaving employee, it is necessarily "back to square one" in addressing the person's behavior.

Conclusion

As long as laws and rules continue to take precedence over morals and values, claims and lawsuits will continue to proliferate. Therefore, it is unlikely that organizations will ever be able to fully protect themselves against wrongful termination claims. However, the progressive disciplinary process provides considerable protection when properly applied. The charges most frequently cited in claims of unjust termination involve discrimination, misrepresentation of facts, absence of due process, lack of evidence, lack of proper warnings, insufficient time to correct the problem, and lack of proper notice of the seriousness of the offense. Nevertheless, despite the multitude of accusations that angry former employees are capable of generating, employers can take comfort in the knowledge that progressive discipline, when consistently applied in a nonretaliatory and nonpunitive manner and completely documented, the relative merit of every charge, complaint, or counterrationale is weakened or altogether negated.

Questions for Review and Discussion

1. Under what kinds of behavioral circumstances do you believe that the full use of all steps in the progressive disciplinary process over time would be appropriate?
2. Explain the primary purpose of progressive discipline and identify some circumstances when it is most likely inappropriate.
3. What is the value of the suspension step in the progressive disciplinary process?
4. Identify and describe one alternative to traditional progressive discipline.
5. Give two examples of situations in which immediate discharge is appropriate and explain why this is so.
6. Why is it necessary that an oral warning be documented?
7. How might an organization go about defending itself against a charge of unjust discharge? Should every such charge be fought?

8. Why do some managers fail to discipline when they should or to the extent that they should?

9. What is the ultimate purpose of documentation of all disciplinary processes?

10. Why is progressive discipline sometimes seen as inappropriate behavior modification?

References

1. Smith, S., & Mazin, R. (2004). *The HR answer book: An indispensable guide for managers and human resource professionals*. New York: American Management Association.
2. Muchinsky, P. (2006). *Psychology applied to work*. Belmont, CA: Thomson Wadsworth.
3. Franklin, A. L., & Pagan, J. F. (2006). Organization culture as an explanation for employee discipline practices. *Review of Public Personnel Administration, 26*(1), 52–73.
4. Skinner, B. F. (1953). *Science and human behavior*. New York: Macmillan.
5. Bernardi, L. (1996). Progressive discipline: Effective management tool or legal trap? *Canadian Manager, 21*(4), 9.
6. Koen, C. M., Jr., & Mitchell, M. S. (2010, January). Supervisor's checklist for termination/discipline. *SuperVision, 27*(1), 3–6.
7. Sundel, M., & Sundel, S. (1999). *Behavioral change in the human services: An introduction to principles and applications* (4th ed.). Thousand Oaks, CA: Sage Publications.
8. Liberman, A., & Rotarius, T. M. (1999). Behavioral contract management: A prescription for employee and patient compliance. *Health Care Manager, 18*(2), 1–10.
9. Robinson, S. L., & Rousseau, D. M. (1994). Violating the psychological contract: Not the exception but the norm. *Journal of Organizational Behavior, 15*, 245–259.
10. Muhl, C. J. (2001, January). The employment-at-will doctrine: Three major exceptions. *Monthly Labor Review*. Available at: www.bls.gov. Accessed August 28, 2009.

Chapter 9

Statutory Benefits: How They Involve the Manager

Robert R. Kulesher, PhD, MHA, BA, *Assistant Professor, Health Services and Information Management, College of Allied Health Sciences, East Carolina University, Greenville, North Carolina*

Chapter Objectives

- Identify and describe the few forms of employee benefits that are mandated by law for all employers and employees, specifically Social Security, Workers' Compensation, unemployment insurance, and short-term disability insurance.
- Differentiate true statutory benefits from other employee benefits that have had their origins in federal legislation.
- Review the principal characteristics and requirements of these statutory benefits.
- Describe how and to what extent the healthcare manager can influence the cost and utilization of those benefits over which some degree of control may be exercised, specifically for Workers' Compensation and unemployment compensation.

Legally Mandated Benefits

There are a number of employee benefits for which neither employer nor employee has the opportunity to opt in or out of participation. As dictated by both state and federal governments, these few benefits are mandated, that is, required by law (statute), so are thus referred as statutory benefits. Essentially everyone who earns a living in a legally constituted work organization is a covered participant under statutory benefits.

The principal statutory benefits that apply to all managers and nonmanagers alike are Social Security, Workers' Compensation, unemployment insurance, and, in a number of states, short-term disability insurance.

There are of course some additional benefits that may appear on the surface to be required by statute. For example, some will doubtless consider the provisions of the Family and Medical Leave Act (FMLA) and Consolidated Omnibus Budget Reconciliation Act (COBRA) to represent statutory benefits.[1] The same might be said of the Americans with Disabilities Act (ADA) and certain other employment-related legislation. Employers are required to abide by these acts under varying circumstances and conditions. For FMLA to be required is determined by the size of an organization (number of employees); for COBRA to be required, the employer had to have been offering health insurance as a benefit, which is an employee option with a great many employers. (FMLA is addressed at length in Chapter 3 and ADA is explored in Chapter 4.)

What differentiates the benefits addressed in this chapter from others such as FMLA and ADA is the complete absence of a participation option. An employee can, for example, elect to access the benefits available under the FMLA or decline to do so; there is nothing in law that states an employee *must* participate in this benefit. But true statutory benefits are essentially mandated for both employer and employee. Employer and employee must both pay taxes to support Social Security; they have no choice in the matter. Employers must provide Workers' Compensation coverage, must pay for unemployment insurance, and, in some states, must provide for short-term disability coverage. Employees automatically become covered under these benefits when they accept employment; there is no option involved.

Statutory benefits impact managers both directly and indirectly according to the size and complexity of the organization and the level of authority and responsibility of the manager. The number of employees a manager supervises, the nature of the work, and the corporate culture of the organization all determine how statutory benefits impact the manager's role in maintaining an effective work environment.

The three most common statutory benefits are Workers' Compensation, unemployment insurance, and Social Security. These benefits arose from social programs originally implemented during the Great Depression of the 20th century. Their intent was simple: Provide employees with economic protection against injury at the workplace and unplanned unemployment, and to provide a measure of security in old age. The employer bears part or all of the cost of these benefits.[2]

Workers' Compensation

Workers' Compensation is a program that provides benefits for employees injured on the job. It is governed by state laws, so requirements vary considerably from state to state. It is a no-fault insurance system that provides wage replacement, medical, and rehabilitation benefits to employees who are injured at work. By participating in state-mandated Workers' Compensation insurance, the employer cannot be held liable for injury to employees. In turn, employees forfeit their right to sue the employer for contributing to the accident or illness that occurred in the course of the employee's work.[1]

Employers have less control over the cost of Workers' Compensation insurance than they have over health insurance costs. Workers' Compensation benefits are an entitlement extended as a condition of employment, and employers must pay the entire cost. State legislatures in many states set the level of benefits paid to injured workers. State insurance commissions regulate the premiums that private insurers may charge to cover these benefits.[3]

Employers meet their obligation to provide Workers' Compensation insurance by purchasing coverage from private insurance companies or state-run insurance funds or by self-insuring. This benefit is unique in comparison with other forms of social insurance as it is prefunded in anticipation of future benefit payments.

There are five types of Workers' Compensation claims:[4]

- Medical-only claims
- Temporary total disability
- Permanent partial disability
- Permanent total disability
- Death

Employer Concerns

The cost of Workers' Compensation is a major concern of the employer. This type of insurance is experience-rated, so it pays for the employer to keep the number of injuries and claims to a minimum. When this can be done through safety programs and employee education, all parties benefit. However, all injuries must be reported, properly addressed, and seen through to their conclusion.

Of recent concern has been the broadening of the definition of what constitutes a work-related injury or disease. When the injury is clearly physical and the cause and effect are immediate, there is little problem. However, there are an increasing number of claims for mental and emotional injury as well as claims for which the time lag between incident or other cause and the emergence of the disease or other result may be measured in years.

What the Manager Can Do to Keep Costs Under Control

- Be proactive in maintaining a safe work area. Consult with risk management and with safety engineers as necessary.
- Follow procedures for documenting and reporting employee accidents, injury, and illness.
- Insist that an appropriate accident report or incident report be generated as soon as possible following each event.

- Review every claim to see if the injury arose out of and was in the course of employment.
- Identify potentially false claims.

A department manager is in the best position to question the validity of a Workers' Compensation claim. The manager knows the duties of each position and the incumbent's job description, and is in a position to know the most common injuries that could occur during such work. Low back pain, for example, is a common complaint of hospital employees whose work requires lifting and moving patients. Therefore, the employment interview process and the organization's preemployment physical examination will address a job applicant's ability to handle a certain amount of weight. An appropriate job description can show the employee what is expected at work and can thus help to reduce injury claims.

In evaluating a claim for an illness or injury be suspicious of the following circumstances:[5]

- A claim is filed for an incident that happened some time ago.
- A claim is originated by a new employee.
- Injuries sustained seem to be inconsistent with the reported cause.
- Injuries sustained appear unlikely given the employee's normal job duties.
- An injury is claimed for which there are no witnesses.
- A claim is filed following a negative performance appraisal or when a planned reduction in force (layoff) is announced.

It is especially important for the manager to attempt to determine that each claim filed truly arose from the claimant's employment. One of the most commonly encountered forms of Workers' Compensation fraud consists of an employee's claim that an injury suffered outside of work actually occurred on the job. Such false claims are driven by money; in terms of replacement of a portion of lost income, Workers' Compensation is far more generous than most short-term disability plans.

Also, the manager is advised to maintain a departmental file on each employee, to contain notes documenting incidents or accidents, instances of tardiness, unplanned absences from work, unprofessional behavior at work, and the like. (Such a file, however, should also include positives such as recognition or commendation from the manager and others.) Many anecdotal notes need not become part of a permanent record unless they figure in some specific following action or occurrence. However, even though a manager's personal files may be thought to be just that—personal—it is advisable to keep all such notes factual and free from subjective judgments. Such a personal file can always be called upon in the event of a legal challenge, so it is best to remember that under certain circumstances, whatever one writes about an employee can conceivably "go public" someday.

Much harder to quantify than physical injuries are claims that arise from job-related stress. A well-documented progressive discipline process may help to combat this kind of claim. Good documentation should detail counseling meetings, recommended training and education, and behavior modification efforts.

In all work areas, inherent hazards should be highlighted at orientation to the department, identified with signage, and regularly discussed at department meetings.

Unemployment Insurance

Unemployment insurance, also referred to as unemployment compensation, came into being along with the establishment of Social Security. The program provides unemployment benefits to eligible workers who become unemployed through no fault of their own and meet other eligibility requirements of state law. Benefits are intended to provide temporary financial assistance to unemployed workers. Individual states are free to set their own limits on weekly benefit amounts, unemployment tax rates, taxable wage bases, and individual eligibility and disqualification requirements. Each state administers its own unemployment insurance program within guidelines established by federal law. Eligibility for unemployment compensation, benefit amounts, and the length of time benefits are available are determined by the state law under which unemployment insurance claims are established. In the majority of states, benefit funding is based solely on a tax imposed on employers. Unemployment insurance is financed by taxing employers a percentage of the annual wages of their employees. The tax is paid to state and federal unemployment compensation funds. The percentage paid by each employer is based on the historical number of claims filed by workers.[1, 6]

Coverage and Eligibility

All workers are covered by the provisions of unemployment insurance except for some agricultural and domestic workers. However, in order to be eligible upon becoming unemployed, a worker must:[2]

- Be able, available, and seeking work;
- Have not refused suitable work;
- Not be unemployed because of a labor dispute;
- Have not left the job voluntarily;
- Have not been terminated for gross misconduct; and
- Have been employed in a covered industry and earned a designated minimum amount for a certain period of time.

The purpose of unemployment compensation is to stabilize personal and regional economies by:[7]

- Providing weekly income during periods of involuntary unemployment such as layoffs and employer closures;

- Stabilizing the economy during recessions;
- Providing employers with the incentive to stabilize their employment; and
- Helping unemployed workers find jobs.

Under most applicable laws, employees who are discharged for cause or who voluntarily resign are not eligible for unemployment compensation. However, some employees who are not eligible nevertheless file claims; filing costs the employee nothing more than a brief visit to the local office of the state employment service. It is essential for the manager—and the organization's administration and human resources function—to appreciate that, in many instances, the undeserving individual will be granted unemployment compensation *unless the employer actively challenges the claim.*

The employer can challenge any unemployment compensation claim, and the departing employee can likewise challenge the employer's unwillingness to concede the claim. A challenge by either employer or employee entitles either party to take the issue to a hearing with the nearest office of the state's employment commission. More often than not, the employer's success at disputing the claim of an individual who has been discharged for cause depends on documentation establishing that the institution's disciplinary process has been properly, objectively, and consistently applied. The necessity for proper documentation, especially all disciplinary steps taken, cannot be overemphasized. The view customarily taken by officialdom of the absence of documentation is if an alleged infraction is not documented, it is assumed to have never happened.

Unemployment benefits are based on a percentage of an individual's earnings over a recent 52-week period up to some maximum amount determined by the state. Benefits can be paid for a maximum of 26 weeks in most states. Extended benefits are often made available during periods of high unemployment. Benefits are subject to federal income taxes and so must be reported as taxable income.

Cost Control

The compensation paid to terminated employees who receive unemployment benefits is charged against the employer. Such charges increase the cost of unemployment insurance to the employer, so it is in the organization's best interest to ensure only legitimate claims are approved. A further and more positive approach is to reduce turnover within the organization. Many of the elements of the cost of terminating an individual may be wholly or partially hidden, but the total cost of any single termination is significant. Thus, programs of intervention before termination, as well as other efforts to reduce unwanted turnover, are necessary and worthwhile.

What the Manager Can Do

Application of the best method for reducing unemployment compensation claims begins before employment with careful applicant screening. Next follows the proper use of a probationary period to further evaluate the abilities of each new employee. The probationary period provides the manager with opportunities to train and evaluate each new employee, culminating in any of the following actions:

- Promoting the new employee from probationary to regular status if probation is successfully completed;
- Extending probation and implementing additional training and education if the employee is showing progress but is "not quite there yet";
- Removing the employee from that particular job and considering placement in some other capacity, if available; and
- Releasing the individual from employment.

Concerning the final point mentioned, releasing from employment an individual who does not successfully complete the probationary period is not to be considered as discharge for cause. Such a separation is not disciplinary; that is, it is not related to employee conduct. It is performance related; the terminated individual did not pass probation, and was thus unable to perform consistent with the requirements of the job. Termination for failure to pass probation is to be treated more as a layoff rather than as termination for cause.

A key point for every manager to remember is that it is far easier and much less legally risky to release an unsuitable employee at the end of probation than to only find it necessary to release the person after regular employee status has been granted. Also, the manager should never advance an unsuitable employee from probation to regular status out of fear of causing a charge of discrimination.

Social Security

Social Security, originally established by law in 1935, has been expanded in scope a number of times over the years. The original legislation and its subsequent amendments established a system of social insurance coverage including retirement income, disability income, survivor income, and health insurance benefits through Medicare. Funding for Social Security is presently 12.4% of an employee's pay up to a gross income ceiling of $106,800. The 12.4% tax is shared equally by employer and employee. Self-employed individuals pay a full 12.4%. As far as this tax is concerned, the self-employed individual is both employer and employee. The foregoing percentages are subject to increase (they have never been known to decrease) by act of the US Congress.

The deduction for Social Security on a payroll receipt appears beside the acronym FICA, OASDI, or the words Social Security. FICA stands for the Federal Insurance Contributions Act. The employer must withhold the aforementioned portion of an employee's salary each pay period and must match the employee's amount and submit the funds to a government account known as the Social Security Trust Fund.

OASDI is the acronym for Old Age, Survivors, and Disability Insurance, the program governing the collection of revenues and distribution of payments under the operative title Social Security.[8]

There is also presently a deduction equivalent to 2.9% of an employee's total earnings (there is no income ceiling) intended for funding Medicare, this deduction being shared equally by employer and employee at 1.45% each. As with the FICA tax, self-employed individuals pay the full amount. The deduction for Medicare on a paycheck receipt may usually be found next to the words Medicare or Hospital Insurance.[1]

Individuals must accumulate a certain number of credits to be eligible for Social Security benefits. The number needed depends on one's age and the type of benefit for which one is applying. A worker can earn a maximum of four credits each year; most individuals need 40 credits to qualify for retirement benefits.

Social Security and Medicare benefits are the least likely to impact the healthcare manager's role. There is little a manager can do to cause a reduction of benefits to employees other than terminating them or withholding wage increases, moves that are unwise and unethical and, in some instances, probably illegal.

Short-Term Disability

Many employers provide short-term disability coverage. There are, however, five states and one territory (Puerto Rico) that require employers to provide short-term disability benefits for all employees. These entities require employers to provide a specified minimum amount of short-term disability benefits to all employees while they are temporarily disabled. Some states permit insurance companies to provide the coverage; others insist that all coverage be provided by the state and paid for through payroll taxes. Each state's plan and administration is handled differently.[9]

- *California*: Provides payment of 55% of the employee's gross salary up to a maximum of $728 per week, after a 1-week waiting period, for up to 52 weeks.
- *New York*: New York requires employers to provide coverage for employees of 50% of salary after 1 week for up to 26 weeks.
- *New Jersey*: New Jersey's law requires payment of two third of salary after 1 week and payment of benefits for up to 26 weeks. After 3 weeks of disability, the plan goes back and retroactively pays the first week of disability as well.
- *Rhode Island*: Benefits start after 7 days and pay up to 30 weeks. The first week is paid retroactively after 4 weeks of disability. The benefit paid is based on a percentage of one's quarterly earnings over a base period. Rhode Island's program is unusual in that it increases the benefit payable for each of the claimant's dependent children younger than age 18.
- *Hawaii*: Hawaii's disability plan pays 58% of salary after 7 days for up to 26 weeks.[13]

Conclusion

All employers are subject to legally mandated benefits as set forth in state and federal law. These statutory benefits include Social Security, unemployment insurance, and Workers' Compensation. Other benefits include the funding of Medicare through employer contribution and employee payroll deduction, and the continuance of group medical insurance after termination from employment. Of all of these benefits, Workers' Compensation and unemployment compensation have the greatest implications for the healthcare manager. Adherence to well-constituted hiring practices, including interviews, job descriptions, orientation, and proper use of probationary periods, all help the organization reduce the number of claims filed for Workers' Compensation and for unemployment. By maintaining and observing well-documented policies governing grievances and disciplinary actions, the employer can exert a measure of control over unemployment costs. And by strict attention to safety, plus examination of questionable claims, the individual manager can help control the organization's Workers' Compensation costs.

Questions for Review and Discussion

1. What is meant by experience-rated in describing an insurance program? Explain.
2. Why should the manager always seek to verify the time and place of occurrence of an injury reported as a Workers' Compensation claim?
3. Define in your own words a true statutory benefit.
4. Where and how can savings result from a department manager's conscientious oversight of unemployment compensation claims?
5. Would you consider it advantageous to automatically challenge every unemployment compensation claim filed? Why or why not?
6. Why should an employee's failure to pass probation not be considered subject to the organization's disciplinary policy?
7. Where and how can savings be generated by a manager's conscientious monitoring of Workers' Compensation claims?

References

1. Mathis, R. L., & Jackson, J. H. (1997). *Human resource management* (8th ed., pp. 436–440). St. Paul, MN: West Publishing Company.
2. Atchison, T. J., Belcher, D. W., & Thomsen, D. J. (2009). *Internet based benefits & compensation administration*. ERI Economic Research Institute. Available at: www.eridlc.com/onlinetextbook/toc.htm. Accessed June 9, 2010.

3. White, J., & Pyenson, B. (1991). *Employee benefits for small business* (pp. 79–90). New York: Prentice Hall General Reference.

4. Worral, J. D., & Durbin, D. L. (2001). Workers' Compensation insurance. In J. S. Rosenbloom (Ed.), *The handbook of employee benefits: Design, funding and administration* (5th ed.). New York: Richard D. Irwin.

5. Frasco, R. J., & Simmers, J. (1993). *Workers' Compensation abuse: An employer's guide to combating fraud through early intervention investigation* (pp. 53–81). Glendale, CA: Griffin Publishing.

6. Penczak, J. A. (1996). Unemployment benefit plans. In J. D. Mamorsky (Ed.), *Employee benefits handbook* (Vol. 2, pp. 40–41). Boston: Warren, Gorham & Lamont.

7. Rejda, G. E. (2001). State unemployment compensation programs. In J. S. Rosenbloom (Ed.), *The handbook of employee benefits: Design, funding and administration* (5th ed., pp. 557–571). New York: McGraw-Hill.

8. Quible, Z. K. (1996). *Administrative office management: An introduction* (6th ed., p. 282). Upper Saddle River, NJ: Prentice Hall.

9. Chambers, J. (2004, June). Short term disability benefits. *HCV Advocate*. Available at: http://www.hcvadvocate.org/hepatitis/hepC/Short_term_DB.html. Accessed February 18, 2010.

Chapter 10

Lawsuit: So You Have to Go to Court

Susie T. Harris, PhD, MBA, RHIA, CCS, *Assistant Professor, Health Services and Information Management, East Carolina University, Greenville, North Carolina*

Chapter Objectives

- Introduce the structure and purpose of the federal and state court systems as they apply to the handling of various legal actions, and review the forms of legal documents that are used to initiate various steps in the legal process.
- Develop an understanding of the legal process of "discovery," including deposition testimony and document production.
- Provide guidelines for healthcare managers who may be required to provide deposition testimony relative to a lawsuit involving medical issues or employment matters.
- Impart knowledge of what the manager may expect if called upon to provide deposition testimony or testify during a court proceeding.

Background

The two court systems operating in the United States are the *state court* and the *federal court*. Both the state and federal systems have explicit duties to perform and specific missions to pursue. A duty may be *exclusive* in that only one particular court system can hear a case, or *concurrent*, in that both court systems have the authority to hear a case. If both systems have jurisdiction to hear a particular case, the plaintiff decides on the court system in which the case will be heard. In criminal cases, the type of crime and the locale where the crime occurred determine where the case will be heard. In civil cases, the court system used depends on the location of the event and the type of lawsuit under consideration.

According to Fremgen, "The federal court system has jurisdiction, or power, to hear a case, when one of the following conditions is present:

- The dispute is related to a federal law or the US Constitution.
- The US government is one of the parties involved in the dispute.
- Different states' citizens are involved in the dispute and the case involves more than $75,000.
- Citizens of another country are involved in a dispute with a US citizen and the case involves more than $75,000.
- The actual dispute occurred in international waters."[1]

If the case does not involve any of the foregoing situations, it must be heard by a state court. Also, unless Congress prohibits state courts from hearing a particular type of case (e.g., a kidnapping that occurs across state lines), the case may still be heard in a state court. All bankruptcy law and patent law cases must be heard in federal court. All divorce, child custody, and probate cases must be heard in state court.

The federal court and state court systems are divided into three levels with cases first being heard at the trial court level. If there is an appeal, the court at the next level will hear the case.

Federal court levels are US District Courts (trial courts), US Courts of Appeals, and finally, the US Supreme Court. State courts are established by the laws of each state and generally follow an arrangement similar to the federal courts, with trial courts, an intermediate appeals court, and the state's highest court typically called the Supreme Court. The names given to these courts vary among the states.

Common Types of Legal Documents

The most common types of legal documents are the subpoena, court order, warrant, deposition notice/subpoena, interrogatories, and request for production. In the context of legal proceedings, medical records are viewed as business records.[2]

Subpoena

According to Pozgar, "A subpoena is a legal order requiring the appearance of a person or the presentation of documents to a court or administrative body." The service of a subpoena at a specified time in advance of the requested appearance (e.g., at least 48 hours) is specified by the jurisdiction.[3] Subpoenas issued by attorneys do not carry the same significance as court orders or court-issued subpoenas. Nevertheless, healthcare providers are obligated to act in response to such requests.[2]

States have different laws that govern subpoenas. For example, in North Carolina, healthcare providers are governed by subpoenas issued by a state court or administrative agency, or a federal court located within 100 miles of the location where the witness is required to appear, or the 4th Circuit Court of Appeals.[2]

A subpoena requires the person(s) named in the document to appear to testify or produce specified documents. Health information managers usually handle two types of subpoenas: a subpoena to testify and a subpoena to produce documents or objects. Other managers (e.g., administrators or managers of human resources) may be required to supply documentation of relevance in employment-related cases.

The subpoena to testify is a written order signed by a judicial official, an attorney, or a party to the action, which commands an individual to appear as a witness in a pending legal action. A subpoena to testify may be served by giving a written copy to the person subpoenaed or by having a sheriff, deputy sheriff, or coroner telephone the person to be subpoenaed. This subpoena requires the person to appear at a court proceeding to testify. It does not require the individual to bring any records, and, in fact, a healthcare manager subpoenaed should not take any patient information when required to testify.[2] *Subpoena ad testificatum* is used interchangeably with subpoena to testify.[4]

Subpoena Duces Tecum

A subpoena to produce documents or objects or a *subpoena duces tecum* "is a written order signed by a judicial official or an attorney that orders an individual with custody of patient information to produce specific documents at a certain time and place, but does not authorize disclosure of the information."[2] In some jurisdictions, it may otherwise be referred to as a notice to produce.

A *subpoena duces tecum* is a written court order requiring a person to appear in court, give testimony, and bring the particular records, files, books, or information as described in the subpoena. The court issues a subpoena for records that document patient care and, in some instances, billing and insurance records. The purpose of issuing a subpoena for a patient's medical record is to receive written evidence of the patient's medical condition and the care that was received.

If the case involves employment matters rather than medical issues, say, for example, that a present or former employee has brought a charge of discrimination against the organization, the records demanded may include personnel files, job descriptions, compensation records, work schedules, and whatever other business records may be considered potentially relevant to the case.

All copying costs associated with subpoenaed records must be borne by the attorney requesting the subpoena. A local sheriff or federal marshal often serves a subpoena, but many state statutes allow anyone over the age of 18 to serve a subpoena. The subpoena may be served either by certified mail or in person, depending on the state requirement.[1] With regard to a grand jury subpoena, no probable cause is required, unlike subpoenas used in other criminal investigations.[4]

A failure to respond when a subpoena to testify has been issued or to produce appropriate documents when a *subpoena duces tecum* has been issued will cause the requesting authority to seek a judicial order forcing testimony or production. A failure to respond to a judicial order issued by a grand jury could end up as contempt of court punishable by jail time until the end of the grand jury's investigation. Also, failing to tell the truth to the jury may result in a separate charge of obstruction of justice or perjury.[4]

Court Order

When a court order has been issued, the disclosure of patient records without the patient's written authorization is approved by the Health Insurance Portability and Accountability Act (HIPAA). Healthcare managers should be aware that a valid court order must (1) be signed by a judge or magistrate, and (2) have the names of the persons listed who are to appear in sequence and testify or produce particular documents. Health information management staff should be compliant with the provisions of the court order.[2]

Warrant

According to the North Carolina Health Information Management Association's Legal Manual, a warrant is a document issued by a court that authorizes the search of a person or place or authorizes the arrest of a person.[2]

Deposition Notice/Subpoena

A deposition is a discovery procedure used to obtain information prior to the actual trial of a case. It consists of an oral examination with questions relating to the matter at issue. It is made under oath and is recorded and transcribed for presentation or at the trial as deemed necessary. Deposition notices are sent out in advance of the deposition to notify the person of the time and place of the deposition. If an individual who is called is not a party to the case, a subpoena must be issued to compel the person to appear for the deposition.[2]

Interrogatories and Requests for Production

Interrogatories are sets of written questions served by one party on another party, to be answered in writing. The purpose of an interrogatory is to provide information to the requesting party for evaluating aspects of the case or to aid in preparation for the trial. An interrogatory answer may be used as evidence during a trial. Requests for production ask for the production of documents in response to specific descriptions.[2]

Tips for Depositions and Trials

In our extremely litigious culture, it behooves most healthcare professionals to be prepared to supply deposition testimony as necessary, testify in court when called upon, or both.

A deposition is part of the fact-finding process. It is sometimes held soon after a lawsuit has been filed, but this is not always so. The pace at which many cases proceed is often largely dependent on the schedules and priorities of the attorneys involved. Since the majority of lawsuits are settled out of court, depositions are highly significant.[5] It is important to know how to prepare for and behave during a deposition or trial. Therefore, the remainder of this chapter offers tips for healthcare managers who are subpoenaed.

Discovery Process

Often months before a trial or hearing is scheduled, lawyers use their rights to force the opposing attorneys to reveal information about a case. The attorneys for the plaintiff and defendant use a variety of methods and tools to gather information.[5] The discovery process involves investigating facts and allegations before the trial.[3]

The objectives of the discovery process are to

> 1) obtain evidence that might not be obtainable at the time of trial; 2) isolate and narrow the issues for trial; 3) gather knowledge of the existence of additional evidence that may be admissible at trial; and 4) obtain leads to enable the discovering party to gather further evidence.[3]

Rules for the discovery process are designed to avoid "trial by ambush." These rules have been established in order for individuals to know the names and addresses of all possible witnesses on the opposing side.[3] Each side is entitled to know who will be appearing on behalf of the other side; the surprise witness is largely a fiction perpetuated by television courtroom dramas.

Methods and tools used in the discovery process are briefly described as follows:

1. Interrogatories (as noted earlier) are "detailed sets of questions that the plaintiff's attorney can compel defendants and witnesses to respond to, in writing."

2. Relevant documents include "the medical record, nurses' notes, and other written materials detailing the plaintiff's care" or personnel files and other business records as appropriate.

3. Incident reports "are typically intended for in-house quality assurance purposes and should not be referenced in the medical record, may be off limits

to a plaintiff's attorney—at least in some states." However, in some states, they may be used as proof in a lawsuit.

4. Depositions are "usually initiated by the plaintiff's attorney in a medical malpractice case"[5] as well as in an employment-related case, although the defendant's attorneys are entitled to depose the plaintiffs if so desiring.

According to textbooks and legal scholars, the purpose of a deposition is fact-finding. However, depositions also serve another purpose: the attorneys on each side, the plaintiff's and defendant's sides, will use a deposition as an opportunity to assess your strengths, weaknesses, appearance, and presentation with respect to how a jury may perceive your testimony.[6]

"Depositions are part of an intensive effort to find out in advance what the witnesses and defendants can be expected to say . . . if the case goes to trial."[5] In a deposition, your testimony gives the other side an opportunity to look for ways to cast doubt upon what you say. Additionally, unlike an actual trial, the attorney who examines the witnesses is allowed to ask leading questions. Your testimony will be recorded and possibly videotaped. However, your deposition testimony usually is not admissible in court unless you are unable to testify at the trial or your testimony in the deposition conflicts with statements in the trial. In summary, it is doubtful that your side will gain anything positive from the deposition. Therefore, you should note that "the less said, the better."[5]

You should expect that the opposing attorney will try to catch you "off guard" by possibly smirking or laughing at something in the testimony or by attempting to win you over by flattery. In either case, you should remain on guard.

The following tips should be kept in mind for a deposition:

1. Listen carefully.
2. Ask for clarification (as many times as needed).
3. Do not volunteer any information.
4. Stay calm.
5. Watch your words.

Being aware of the pitfalls of a deposition should assist you in ensuring that your testimony precisely addresses the issue at hand. Gart suggests that you review other depositions and also go through a mock deposition prior to testifying in an actual deposition.[7]

Lisa A. Miller, CNM, JD, a certified midwife and attorney, recommends 10 rules for surviving a deposition while "swimming with the sharks."

1. Don't take it personally.
2. Make the medical record your best friend.
3. Be actively involved in your defense.
4. Listen carefully and answer only what is asked.

5. Take your time.

6. Know your stuff.

7. Realize that "I don't know" and "I don't recall" are acceptable, yet distinctly different answers.

8. Leave out your opinions.

9. Excuse yourself as needed.

10. Don't take it personally.[6]

You should approach a deposition with confidence; that is, minus any visible signs of uneasiness or reluctance if you can possibly do so. Beware, however, of overconfidence that can manifest itself in a noticeable casual or "flip" attitude and never, never try to be funny. Also, keep in mind that you are responsible for providing factual information in a deposition. In this capacity, you are what is referred to as *fact witness*, you are not an *expert witness*. Before the deposition date, your organization's attorney should brief you concerning what to expect. And whether suggested or not, you should review all the documents available to help prepare yourself for the deposition. You may be asked during the deposition what documents you have reviewed. However, do not write anything down because any document you create may be subpoenaed.[8]

Once you enter the room where the deposition will be held, experts suggest these useful guidelines:

1. "Tell the truth. This is the fundamental, unbreakable rule of testifying at a deposition or in court. Answer every question truthfully. If you don't know the answer, say so. If you don't remember what happened—and memories do fail during what can be years between incidents and depositions—say so. Attorneys are trained to pick up on false testimony, and they are trained to ask the same questions in multiple ways to uncover discrepancies in your answers. If the case goes to court, any discrepancies in your testimony will be used in attempts to discredit you. . . Fooling an attorney is difficult, so don't try."[8] If you are asked your opinion, you can say, "I'm a fact witness, not an expert witness."[8]

2. "Be brief. Many questions can be answered with a simple 'yes' or 'no.' Do not launch into a 20-minute dissertation on an incident. Just respond with a direct answer focused on the specific question."[8]

3. Be prepared to defend yourself. Attorneys may question your credentials and every aspect of your work related to the matter that is the subject of the lawsuit. Stay calm and defend yourself. Make reference to employer, professional, or industry standards, policies, or procedures that support you.

4. Speak in plain language. Your role in a deposition is to educate attorneys—and, in a trial, judges and juries—about medical technology or other matters in which your listeners are not well versed. Like any specialist, you

may use technical terms or acronyms to talk about equipment in everyday interactions. In a deposition, though, even highly educated attorneys may not understand you. Use common analogies and plain language to explain how things work.

5. Slow down and take a breath. Walking into a deposition room can be a daunting experience. There may be a number of attorneys representing various parties to the lawsuit, all of them ready to question you. It is suggested that you take a breath before you say anything, then talk slowly—this gives your attorney time to object to an issue or question."[8]

Expert Witnesses

Physicians, nurses, and other professionals are often called to serve as expert witnesses in court cases. Courts depend on expert witnesses in most civil and criminal cases to clarify and explain certain matters that may not be understood by jurors and judges. For example, an expert witness can evaluate the pertinent standards of care with the essentials of the case in question and infer whether or not the facts indicate a digression from applicable standards of care.[9]

Professionals within your own organization may be set forth as experts to give weight to the testimony that you and others who are called may offer. However, a great many expert witnesses are paid participants hired by the opposing sides, resulting in often conflicting testimony by the defendant's expert versus the plaintiff's expert. It is relatively common to find that the "experts" engaged in a case are not in agreement. Understandably, each side will engage only paid "experts" who will testify in support of or in agreement with the hiring side's position. It is then left to judge or jury to decide which testimony seems most credible.

Witness Preparation

The way in which a witness handles questioning during a trial or deposition is critical to the case. In fact, it is frequently as significant as the facts of the case. Being well prepared before testifying in a trial or deposition should be the goal of a witness. Pozgar offers these guidelines to follow in order to be well prepared to testify:

1. Review the records (e.g., medical records and other business records) about what you might be questioned.

2. Do not be antagonistic in answering questions. The jury may already be somewhat sympathetic toward a particular party to the lawsuit; antagonism may only serve to reinforce such an impression.

3. Be organized in your thinking and recollection of the facts regarding the incident.

4. Answer only the questions asked.

5. Explain your testimony in simple, succinct terminology.

6. Do not overdramatize the facts you are relating.

7. Do not allow yourself to become overpowered by the cross-examiner.

8. Be polite, sincere, and courteous at all times.

9. Dress appropriately and be neatly groomed.

10. Pay close attention to any objections your attorney may have to the line of questioning being conducted by the opposing counsel.

11. Before appearing as a witness, be sure to review the record of any deposition in which you may have participated during earlier phases of the case.

12. Be straightforward with the examiner. Any answers designed to cover up or cloud an issue or fact will, if discovered, serve only to discredit any previous testimony that you may have given.

13. Do not show any visible signs of displeasure regarding testimony with which you are in disagreement.

14. Be sure to ask to have questions that you did not hear repeated and questions that you did not understand rephrased.

15. If you are not sure of an answer, indicate that you are not sure or that you do not know the answer.[3]

One final bit of emphasis relative to your appearance before your questioners: Whether giving deposition testimony or testifying at a trial, be thoroughly professional. Appear professional and behave professionally. Your overall appearance and demeanor may well affect your credibility.

Conclusion

After a lawsuit is filed, there may be early offers of settlement. However, if either side believes that it has a case of sufficient strength, early settlement is unlikely and matters will proceed to the discovery phase. During discovery, depositions are likely, as are demands for the production of documents. Anywhere throughout the total process, there may be settlement terms offered or asked for. At this stage, it is not unusual for a defendant organization to agree to a settlement simply to avoid the expense and disruption of a trial. Lacking settlement and following completion of discovery, the case may go to trial.

Healthcare managers are advised to follow the guidelines provided in this chapter in preparing for the important once- or twice-in-a-lifetime experience of testifying at a deposition or at trial.

Questions for Review and Discussion

1. Why should it be necessary to respond to deposition questions if most of the same questions may be asked during trial?

2. Why are you advised to volunteer nothing when being deposed, even when you feel you have something important to add?

3. If expert witnesses on opposing sides of a case provide contradictory testimony, what is the value of having experts at all?

4. What would you do if the plaintiff's attorney in a lawsuit legally requests documentation that runs into hundreds or thousands of pages?

5. When does a plaintiff have some choice as to whether his or her case is heard in a state court or a federal court?

6. What will be your reaction if you are being deposed and the attorney asks a lengthy question that is actually two or three questions in one?

7. What are the fundamental differences between a subpoena and a court order?

8. Why might your organization's top management be agreeable to settling a case out of court even though they believe in the rightness of their position?

9. Why are deposition witnesses invariably advised to remain calm even though questioning may become rude and accusatory?

10. Patient records and employee personnel files have long been recognized as confidential documents. How, then, do these documents become a visible part of a lawsuit for any number of strangers to review?

References

1. Fremgen, B. R. (2009). *Medical law and ethics* (3rd ed., p. 361). Upper Saddle River, NJ: Pearson Prentice Hall.

2. North Carolina Health Information Management Association. (2007). *Legal reference manual* (p. 203). Chicago, IL: American Health Information Management Association.

3. Pozgar, G. D. (2004). *Legal aspects of health care administration* (9th ed., p. 560). Sudbury, MA: Jones and Bartlett.

4. Spevak, C. (2006). The grand jury and health care crimes: What every physician executive needs to know. *Physician Executive, 32*(1), 68–70.

5. Di Luigi, K. J. (2004). Giving a deposition? *RN, 67*(1), 63–69.

6. Miller, L. A. (2004). Swimming with sharks: Ten tips for surviving a deposition. *Neonatal Network: The Journal of Neonatal Nursing, 23*(5), 67–69.

7. Gart, M. (2008). Medical malpractice: Deposition. *Physician Executive, 34*(3), 66–68.

8. Vockley, M. (2006). Called to testify? *Biomedical Instrumentation & Technology, 40*(6), 429–434.

9. American Academy of Pediatrics. (2009). Expert witness participation in civil and criminal proceedings. *Pediatrics, 124*, 428–438.

Chapter 11

Ethics and the Manager: Everyday Hazards

Llewellyn E. Piper, PhD, *President and Chief Executive Officer, Onslow Memorial Hospital, Jacksonville, North Carolina*

Chapter Objectives

- Recognize the extent to which potential ethical dilemmas can involve the healthcare manager.
- Review the history and development of ethics.
- Provide working definitions of ethics, morality, and trust.
- Review the critical role of trust in the effective operation of an organization.
- Stress the importance of developing and maintaining a culture of ethics throughout the organization.
- Review the potential ethical hazards faced by the healthcare manager on a regular basis.
- Prepare the manager to recognize where unethical considerations and the law converge, and when what is unethical becomes illegal.

Introduction

Today's healthcare managers are faced with many ethical demands in the fulfillment of their vital mission to serve society with the delivery of quality and safe medical care. Healthcare managers are charged with multiple challenges in managing many resources, including finances, staff, supplies, and equipment, and in planning for and directing the activities of staff. They also are challenged by their colleagues, the organizational mission and culture, and patients and the public. These ethical demands are the reflection of our times; the spirit of the present is defined by a public that questions the ethics of healthcare delivery more than ever. The public today reflects a degree of paranoia and fear where health care is concerned. People are concerned about access to care, and they wonder what could go wrong for them, their families, or their friends as patients. People question the cost and affordability of health care, and they are concerned about how healthcare reform will affect them.

Among the demands on healthcare managers, there is always the question of how to ensure ethical behavior in all that they do. Most managers today act out of good intent but are often confronted with gray ethical areas and fuzzy ethical boundaries. They may also find themselves committing unethical behavior with the intent of assisting friends by "bending the rules" and finding themselves behaving illegally. One might also commit an unethical and illegal act for selfish reasons, such as taking bribes or kickbacks, or committing Medicare or Medicaid fraud. Health care has evolved into the major social safety net of today's society, but there are many circumstances that can place a manager and the organization in breach of both ethical behavior and the law.

In today's society, not a day goes by without some significant ethical violations occurring on the national, state, or local scene. From the ubiquitous criminal acts of murder, robbery, rape, and gang violence, to national and international corporate fraud and financial and banking crises reflecting failures of trust, to questioning the morality of numerous highly placed office holders, the ethical barriers of morality and trust seem constantly breached. From Enron's accounting scandal to the financial collapse of Lehman Brothers and Bernard Madoff's massive Ponzi scheme one can see countless recent examples of how ethics has been grossly compromised and trust has been destroyed.

In health care, there are ethical issues related to the quality and safety of care, credentialing questionable providers, questionable appropriateness of many procedures and tests, and billing fraud. Often the healthcare manager is caught in the middle of such ethical issues.

To appropriately address ethical concerns, it is helpful for today's healthcare manager to know something of the history of ethics and the ways in which ethics, morality, and trust are related. To know how to respond to ethical dilemmas, the manager should also be aware of the more obvious questions of ethical behavior occurring in gray areas in which issues are clouded by circumstances. The manager may often feel trapped between opposing forces in the broad gray zone of the ethical continuum.

For the healthcare manager to gain a better understanding of ethics and how ethics, morality, and trust are related, an overview of the history of ethics is provided.

History

The discourse on ethics is as old as human civilization. From the Greek philosophers, Socrates and Plato, we obtain the basis for the need for and the purpose of ethics. In recorded writings from 400 BC until the present, concern for ethics and for the ability of the human spirit to cope with ethical issues have been ongoing themes in all societies. In human behavior, a strong underlying force driving the ongoing ethics dialogue has always been the tendency for the strong to exploit the weak.[1]

Although Socrates left no writings, we have learned of his thoughts on ethics through his followers and students, of whom Plato is considered the most knowledgeable. Influenced by Socrates's thoughts, Plato devoted himself to exploring ethical questions. Socrates was considered then and still today as one of the wisest thinkers of all time. His method of gaining knowledge was through a dialectic with others concerning their ethical beliefs. Socrates asked people to explore common ethical qualities such as self-control, justice, or courage. He found that those he asked really did not know precisely what was meant by such terms. Socrates believed that if humans knew the true nature of justice, the problems and challenges involved in being ethical would be simple. He spent his entire life in the struggle to achieve truth in his knowledge of ethics. It was through ethics, Socrates believed, that mankind would find justice.[1]

The central theme of Plato's *The Republic* is the hope of achieving justice for society. Plato saw the continuing dialogue about justice as a continuing debate between the two major forces of his time: political power and philosophical power. He believed that mankind would have no relief from adversity until real philosophers gained political power or politicians became true philosophers. Plato decided to abandon a political career soon after Socrates's death to spend his life pursuing ethics as the basis for a society's ability to prevail into perpetuity.[1] *The Republic* concludes with the quote that establishes the continual pursuit of an ethical course driven by the soul for justice.

> We should believe the soul to be immortal, capable of enduring all evil and all good and always keep our feet on the upward way and pursue justice and wisdom. So we shall be at peace with the gods and with ourselves, both in our life here and when, like the victors in the games, collecting their prizes, we receive our reward; and both in this life and in the thousand-year journey which I have described, all will be well with us.[1]

The history of Roman society teaches us about ethics as carried over from Greek thinkers such as Socrates and Plato. The Roman Empire provides a lesson in ethical behavior that is paramount to the longevity of a society. The downfall of Rome is relevant today in the continuing struggle with ethical issues. A sound perspective on the ethics of Rome is found in the life and times of Marcus Tullius Cicero.

Considered the greatest statesman of ancient Rome and perhaps of all time, Cicero faced ethical challenges throughout his life as a senator of the Roman Empire. Born around 106 BC, at his father's insistence, Cicero pursued further education in public speaking and the study of law at the age of 16 (the Roman age of majority). He found that he had a gift for writing and public speaking, which served him well as the most famous statesman of all time. He became the voice of ethical conduct for the Roman Empire under the rule of Caesar, who was 6 years younger than Cicero.

Cicero's ethics ultimately triumphed when Caesar was assassinated by Marcus Brutus, one of Cicero's closest friends. For Cicero, the power of ethics could overthrow the excessive and unchecked power of an unethical dictator who had lost sight of the common good of humanity.[2]

About 77 BC, Cicero became a senator in Rome. He viewed a stable society as one that should be in harmony and based on ethical behavior, as reflected in the following quote:

> Just as in the music of harps and flutes or in the voices of singers a certain harmony of the different tones must be maintained . . . so also a state is made harmonious by agreement among dissimilar elements. This is brought about by a fair and reasonable blending of the upper, middle, and lower classes, just as if they were musical tones. What musicians call harmony in song is concord in a state.[2, p. 77]

Cicero's life of resistance to unethical behavior; abuse of power; tyranny; infidelity; financial, legal, and voting corruption; and political agendas of self-interest have been studied by many modern leaders who helped shape the history of Great Britain and the United States, including Queen Elizabeth, Winston Churchill, George Washington, John Adams, Thomas Jefferson, and Abraham Lincoln.[2]

From Christianity, we learn of the plight of Jesus during his short time on earth, calling for moral and ethical behavior for all mankind. We learn from the life of Jesus that one may act with moral and ethical intent to fight evil with good, but that, in the end, evil from an immoral society may sometimes prevail. As stated in the Bible:

> Then the whole company of them arose and brought him before Pilate. And they began to accuse him, saying, "We found this man perverting our nation, and forbidding us to give tribute to Caesar, and saying that he himself is Christ a king" . . . And Pilate said . . . "I find no crime in this man." But they were urgent, saying, "He stirs up the people."[3, p. 81–82]

In *Democracy in America*, the classic treatise on the American way of life written by Alexis De Tocqueville based on his and Gustave de Beaumont's visit to America in 1831, De Tocqueville describes democracy in America as based on the underlying premise of ethical behavior in the equality and trust of the majority.[4] Tocqueville writes, "Amongst the novel objects and that attracted my attention . . . nothing struck me more forcibly than the general equality of condition among the people."[4, p. 11]

Tocqueville saw man's fate as his own, his destiny awaiting his own creation. He saw that nations cannot prevent mankind from achieving equality. He believed that equality depended upon mankind, and that the principle of equality was to lead from servitude to freedom. In America, De Tocqueville believed that with free will and wisdom, people could the see the potential pitfalls of the breach of ethical intent, which, in the extreme, would lead to the subversion of freedom by the tyranny of an unethical majority.[4]

Age-old questions concerning ethics and morality and their role in guiding human behavior remain with us today. Ethics is paramount to the advancement of mankind and is central to justice in the functioning of society. The history of ethics shows that in the constant struggle of good versus evil, good may not always win, but ethics will always be pursued for the betterment of people and society.

Definitions of Ethics, Morality, and Trust

Our definition of ethics arises from the interpretation works of philosophers such as Plato, Kant, and Hume. The term "ethics" is best understood through consideration of how it relates to and is distinguished from morality and trust.

Ethics, as defined in Merriam-Webster's *Collegiate Dictionary*, is "the discipline dealing with what is good and bad and with moral duty and obligation; a set of moral principles or values; the principles of conduct governing an individual or a group; a guiding philosophy."[5]

In *The Republic,* Plato postulated that ethics is all about finding justice for society and for the individual. Plato believed that the best hope for society is found through education, which changes statesmen into philosophers.[1]

Wood states that Kant revolutionized the foundations of philosophical ethics by changing ethics from a science directed toward achieving a pregiven good, or a study of the way human actions and evaluations are controlled by natural sentiments, into an inquiry into the way free agents govern their own lives according to self-given rational principles.[6]

Hume proposed a moral philosophy in the discussion and understanding of ethics. Hume postulated that no action can be virtuous, or morally good, unless there is some motive in human nature. Hume distinguishes a human virtue *as* moral versus a duty *to be* moral. He states that merely doing one's duty is clearly not the same as doing one's duty from a sense of necessity.[7] The sublime essence of human action lies in the question of whether one behaves morally because one wants to or because one is required to.

Hume states, "that deity is the ultimate author of all government and will never be denied by any who strive toward the plans of an Omniscient Being, who can never be deceived by any event or operation."[7, p. 361] Hume believed in an original contract by which subjects have tacitly reserved the power of resisting their sovereign whenever they find themselves aggrieved by that authority.

From a psychological perspective, moral behavior is shaped by one's environment during the early developmental years of life. This moral development concerns rules and conventions concerning what people should do in their interactions with others. Moral behavior is guided by the principles of what is right or wrong within a given society, culture, or setting. Through social learning with reinforcement and punishment, one learns early in life what is and is not acceptable behavior. So a major determinant of one's morality is based on early childhood exposure to what is right and wrong within a given situation. A person's ethical foundation is constructed within the environment of childhood.[8]

Two critical parts of learning moral behavior involve the development of empathy and self-control. Empathy is both an emotional state and a cognitive component, the ability to both react to another person's feelings with an emotional response that is similar to the other person's feelings and to be able to understand the impact of the person's behavior on someone else. In self-control, one learns to self-regulate impulses. Within rigid environments of rights and wrongs, a person becomes conditioned to control impulses, whereas in an environment without guidelines as to what is right and wrong, a person fails to learn self-control and moral behavior.[8]

Several experts offer operational definitions of trust. Fukuyama states that trust is "the expectation that arises within a community of regular, honest, and cooperative behavior, based on commonly shared norms, on the part of other members of that community."[9] Shore writes that, "trust is an unwritten agreement between two or more parties for one party to perform a set of agreed-on activities and for the other party to perform a set of agreed-on activities without fear of change from either party."[10] Covey believes trust means confidence (i.e., when you trust someone, you have confidence in them and in their integrity and abilities).[11]

Simply said, trust means being honest, doing what you say you will do, and being confident in what you do. In healthcare management, we expect that our community will trust us to do our mission and trust that we have the skills, education, and training to accomplish the mission of quality patient care delivery in a safe environment.

Covey sees trust as,

> the one thing that is common to every individual, relationship, team, family, organization, and civilization and if removed will destroy the most powerful government, the most successful organization, the most influential leadership, the greatest friend, the strongest character, the deepest love.[11, p. 5]

For a better understanding of how ethics, morality, and trust connect and operate within the management of a healthcare organization, a model in Figure 11-1 is provided. This model shows that the foundation of leadership and management within a healthcare organization is ethics. Unless a manager is firmly grounded in the values of ethics, nothing else will follow—that is, no development of morality within the organizational culture and no trust within or outside of the organization. Ethics is sublime to all human interaction within a healthcare organization; from it, all positive human interactions founded on the principles of right and wrong are possible.

For a healthcare organization to be competitive and remain able to recruit and retain good staff, it must have values that reflect ethics. The product of an organizational culture of ethics is trust. Trust is powerful; complete trust is the ultimate achievement of any healthcare organization. But trust is difficult to attain, and, once attained, it can be lost in seconds. Trust is difficult to achieve because it is based on total management support of a culture of ethics and morality.

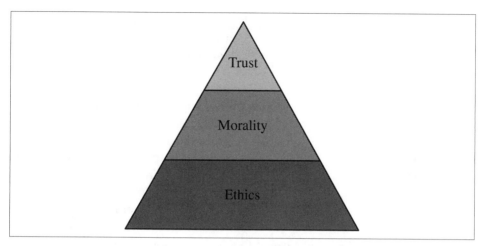

Figure 11-1 *Ethics Model*

Trust is also a human quality to which everyone can relate. It is about the fear of the unknown as it pertains to respect, dignity, and honesty in providing medical diagnoses, assessment, and treatment. The community wants to know that they can trust the healthcare system. People ask: Will I be safe? Will they do me no harm? Will they respect me as an individual and as a human being? Will they respect my confidentiality? Can I trust them with my self or my loved ones?

Nature Versus Nurture

It is natural for humans to develop ethical behavior with moral guidelines and principles and to trust others. By nature, newborns are programmed to learn and to adapt to changing external stimuli. The brain is programmed to support the newborn, prewired to learn from birth about the environment and to adapt for the sake of survival. The driving inborn nature of all humans is to learn how to survive at all costs.[8]

When young, humans are dependent upon the support of others in their environment for survival. Because of this need for nurturing to survive and thrive during the first few years of life, humans become social creatures. At birth, humans are dependent on caregivers for several years for support of basic physiological needs, such as nourishment and fluids. Newborns are also dependent on others for safety from the elements and from harm.[8]

Trusting, learning, and adapting to the rules of the environment create the foundation for ethics, moral behavior, and trust. According to the theory of the great psychosocial developmental psychologist, Erik Erikson, humans develop trust or mistrust within the first 2 years of life based on how one is cared for and loved. According to Freud and supported by psychosocial theorist Erikson and the moral development theorist Kohlberg, humans learn ethics and form a moral code of conduct from their environment based on the rules of behavior. If the environment lacks ethical guidelines to separate right and wrong, the person will grow to adulthood lacking both ethics and a moral conscience and will exhibit a sense of mistrust.[8]

Ethics is based on learning and conditioning in a nurturing environment that provides clearly defined rules of appropriate behavior and the rights and wrongs in adapting and functioning in a social setting. Ethics is a learned value set produced by modeling behavior. Once someone has learned a value set of ethical behavior, this is difficult to change because the individual has learned to survive using the ethical guidelines by which he or she was conditioned to during the early formative years. To develop humans with ethics, one must address the environment in which one developed.[8]

Trust is critical in the development of ethical behavior. Because humans are by nature social beings from the very beginning, infants start out life by trusting others. Through nurturing (or lack thereof), the parent–child bond either supports this trust or the infant will learn to mistrust. Along with the formation of trust or mistrust is the process of learning the rules of right and wrong behavior, as supported by positive or negative reinforcement. These rules form the value set of ethics from which one learns moral or immoral conduct.[8]

There are two models that can assist the healthcare manager in gaining an understanding of ethical behavior. One is the concentric circle model that shows the intent of behavior; the other is the continuum model showing that ethical behavior lies along a continuum.

The concentric model showing intent is shown in Figure 11-2.

As suggested by the model, humans perform at work and pursue their purpose in life based on either the inner circle or the outer circle. In healthcare organizations, those who come from the outer circle are staff members who serve others. They

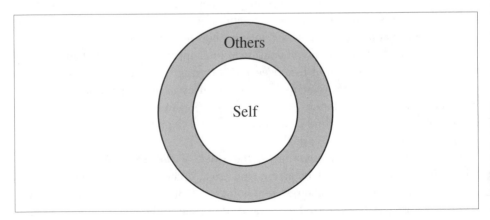

Figure 11-2 *Ethics Behavior Motivation*

follow principles of moral behavior and they have earned the trust of others. They are the solid, committed team members; they comply with organizational rules, policies, and the law. They are loyal, dedicated, and altruistic. They ask: How may I help you? Is there anything I can do for you? They set an ethical example for others in the organization. Based on their ethics, others trust them and they trust others.

Those who come from the inner circle will do whatever it takes to succeed. They follow the rules only if necessary to get what they want. Rules and policies are the only means to a self-serving end. Ethics is not their guideline for performance. They essentially have just two questions: What have you done for me lately? And don't you know that it's all about me? These members of the staff break rules and eventually commit ethical breaches for their own purposes. Often, there arises the challenge for the manager to do what is necessary to discipline and perhaps eventually terminate those who behave unethically. Failure to respond to these inner-circle people will cause the manager to lose trust and become seen as a manager lacking the moral courage to enforce ethical behavior.

Healthcare managers themselves may fall within either circle. Not all managers behave ethically. Some have been able to advance while violating ethics, usually in those questionable gray areas when their behavior may not be sufficiently severe enough to warrant discipline or comprise grounds for legal action or termination. In such cases, the unethical manager perpetuates and validates for the subordinates the belief that unethical behavior is accepted.

To have a culture of ethics, ethical behavior must start at the top within the organization (i.e., from the board), and come through the chief executive officer (CEO) and the managers. Visible ethics can never rise from the bottom up; it is always top down. The board and management must establish ethics within the organization by first behaving ethically themselves and setting the boundaries of what is acceptable and not acceptable. Only then will the individual manager be supported in following through with ethical behavior and acting against unethical behavior.

The continuum mode, shown in Figure 11-3, illustrates how human behavior falls along a continuum from ethical to unethical behavior. This model attempts to address the question: Why do some staff members behave as they do?

All human behavior is driven by either inborn needs, or by wants or desires. Needs are the inborn biological, physiological, psychological, social, and spiritual requirements for human well-being. Wants are those things that create a drive to satisfy some pleasure or desire that is not required for survival or for biological necessity.[8]

+ Mild	Moderate	Severe −
Moral Behavior	Gray Zone	Immoral Behavior

Figure 11-3 *Ethics Continuum*

In satisfying a need or want, a person's behavior falls along an ethical continuum from unethical and immoral to ethical and moral. A person's judgment in behaving in an ethical or unethical perspective is guided by what the person has learned during the early years of development.[8]

In the model in Figure 11-3, behaviors at the unethical and immoral extreme of the continuum are actions that are illegal (i.e., crimes against society). A person who has decided to break the law has, in effect, decided to go against the welfare of the social group and society at large. These extreme behaviors are acts such as homicide, rape, robbery, and fraud, just to mention a few. People who participate in such acts have little or no positive regard for anyone and do not empathize with others; they justify their actions as an exercise of their rights. They will do whatever it takes to get ahead or to support their drive for some personal desire.

The other extreme of the ethical continuum represents ethical and moral behavior. These behaviors represent the highest order of human conduct, driven by a stoic adherence to the rules of ethical behavior. Such members of the healthcare staff know what is right and what is wrong; members of the staff at this end of the ethical continuum always exhibit ethical conduct. Their behavior complies with rules, policies and protocols, and with the law. They are, by nature, altruistic. They believe in serving others and they feel they have a calling that goes beyond them. They do not become absorbed by the inner circle of wants and "What's in it for me?"

The challenge for healthcare managers is in the necessity to properly manage their own behavior and the behavior of their employees when it occurs within a questionable zone—a gray area—of ethical behavior.

Managers may fall into the gray area by the nature of their service to others and by their own need for positive regard for others. In their efforts to please and support others, healthcare managers may find themselves committing minor but questionable acts within the gray area, as shown in Figure 11-3. They may also be unable to detect this type of behavior among their employees because they have become desensitized to this behavior, and begin to view the behavior as acceptable. This paradox of trying to help others can cause managers to breach ethics while remaining unable to recognize their behavior as unethical. They may find they are "caught between."

Everyday Hazards: Caught Between

In the gray zone of the ethical continuum, there is a dilemma that can be referred to as "caught between," the necessity to make a decision that has both positive and negative implications. The manager feels that in making the decision he or she can be doing something that pleases certain others or that condones some situation. Yet, at the same time, the decision maker feels there is something not quiet right but knows that the action is nevertheless supported by top management or has always been considered in the organization as acceptable.

From a psychological perspective, one who is caught between is facing an anxiety of approach-avoidance, double-approach, or double-avoidance. Approach-avoidance occurs, for example, when (1) a friend asks you to go to lunch but the friend is also your employee; (2) you accept a gift for helping a patient and family during care; (3) you write a recommendation for someone who you really believe does not warrant such; and (4) you are asked to support or comment favorably on a decision you dislike but you feel may get you in trouble if you speak the truth. These are a few of the many everyday hazards that can place the manager in the gray zone, caught between wanting to help, to accept, or to decline.

The double-approach occurs when the individual has to lean toward or emphasize one of two competing options. Examples include: (1) going to night school to get a degree while having to work and trying to balance both; (2) balancing child care and work; (3) being required to attend two meetings scheduled at the same time; and (4) choosing to fill a position from two qualified candidates, one of whom is your friend. The anxiety created in the double-approach is that a person wants to wholly support both alternatives, but must choose only one.

Double-avoidance occurs when two undesirable options exist and the manager does not want to support either but is required to support one them. Some examples of these challenges include: (1) you must reduce staff or increase productivity with an already limited staff; (2) you must confront or ignore an employee about an important issue; and (3) you must try to resolve a patient complaint by confronting both the disruptive physician who caused the complaint and the difficult and demanding patient who made the complaint.

Ethical conduct is based not only on what is right, but also on the need for the behavior to be fair and beneficial for all concerned. Behavior is driven by intent; unethical behavior is driven by the intent to benefit oneself at the expense of others, whereas ethical behavior is based on the intent to serve the greater good of all involved.

Unethical behavior not only disregards social rules and values, but also the harm that it may cause oneself, others, and the organization. Unethical behavior is unaccompanied by a sense of remorse or empathy and shows little regard for the rights of others or the organization.

Along the ethical continuum, a healthcare manager is challenged by the dilemma of being caught between and by the need to face the many everyday hazards in the gray zone.

One of the most recognized gray-zone hazards is the post quid quo pro. This occurs when the individual does something that is considered a normal part of the job but is nevertheless rewarded with a gift or other benefit for his or her service. Gifts themselves fall along a continuum from minor to major, from, for example, a restaurant certificate to an expense-paid trip.

Another gray-zone hazard lies in being coerced into doing favors. For example, a neighbor, friend, or family member prevails upon a personal relationship and asks a manager to get someone hired. The manager may be asked to "pull some strings" to get a particular contract approved for a friend, acquaintance, or relative. Perhaps the manager is asked to "buck the line" to get someone an appointment where there is a waiting list. The danger with these favor-hazards is that the manager is not only breaking the rules but is also forcing others to compromise their ethics to support the demands of the manager. A greater hazard lies in the damage these behaviors cause for ethics, morality, and trust within the organization.

Another gray area that plagues managers is the temptation to be less-than-honest under certain circumstances, especially performance evaluations. A manager may like an employee and consider that person a friend, and thus provide a better-than-deserved evaluation to protect the relationship. Or, more unethical by far, the undeserved evaluation is even more likely if there is a sexual relationship involved between manager and employee. Another example includes the overinflated evaluation that may be delivered when the manager does not have the courage to confront an employee whose performance is less than optimal. This practice is also unfair to the employees who have earned good evaluations because giving an undeserved evaluation to an employee whose performance is substandard cheapens the entire evaluation process.

Some managers give in to the temptation to inflate their budgets. In "gaming the system," the manager anticipates that the budget submitted will automatically be cut. If the budget is indeed cut upon submission—meaning the fiscal folks are playing the "game" as well—the manager who submitted the inflated budget may achieve the desired result. If the fiscal folks are indeed "gaming," then managers who have submitted honest budgets may find their budget needs have been reduced. The entire strategy impacts ethical managers, whose budgets may get cut more to support a dishonest manager, and may also harm the overall financial ability of the organization to meet its mission.

There are many ethical hazards in day-to-day management. Managers who get "caught between" and those who live constantly in the gray zone need the attention of top management.

Top management awareness is critical. Leadership must be sensitive to the ethical issues that managers at all lower levels are facing, but once aware of these issues, leadership must provide direction for correction. Failure to correct conditions that are known to provide ethical dilemmas is itself a visible example of unethical behavior, one that sends a powerful and negative message about the organization's culture.

Unique Everyday Hazards for the Manager

Healthcare organizations are essentially unique in the complexity of their mission; this creates unique human interactions that challenge the manager. The complexity exists because of the systems and behaviors required to ensure the quality and safe delivery of services. Every day, these systems and behaviors must accommodate the extremes of demands that range from low-risk to life-and-death situations, from a routine physical exam to stabilizing trauma in the emergency room with open-heart surgery.

Within health care's multiple systems, teams of workers are required to perform in ethical harmony with no agenda other than what is best for the patient. Within these teams is an array of individuals of greatly varied education, experience, and responsibilities. Individual skills, knowledge, and experience range from entry-level workers in services areas to highly skilled medical specialists and the top management of the organization.

In a setting that calls for assessing and treating patients at all levels of care and supervising what is often a mix of professionals and nonprofessionals, managers must balance multiple demands while coping with the unique hazards that present within healthcare organizations.

There are four unique ethical hazards that healthcare managers must face. These can be referred to as the four Ds: (1) drug diversion, (2) documentation in health records, (3) delay of care both intentional and unintentional, and (4) divulging confidential information.

Drug diversion is a hazard for nurses and physicians and others who have access to controlled medications. Some professionals who regularly handle controlled drugs can become so desensitized to handling these substances that they may see no problem in diverting some for their own use. But some of these users become addicted and eventually get caught; at this stage the manager must address the issues related to such unethical and generally illegal behavior.

Documentation in medical records, both in hard copy and electronic form, presents hazards for persons who have access to the records. The ethical breach occurs when someone alters a medical record to cover up a mistake or perhaps divulges a record's contents to persons who have no legitimate need for the information. Some may commit an ethical breach by viewing records for reasons of curiosity or for passing information to others. The staff members who handle records also have the opportunity to alter records to protect themselves from questions of inappropriate care.

Intentional delay of care may arise when someone acts from a passive–aggressive motivation to punish a difficult patient or family member, perhaps someone who has been rude or demanding. Such intentional delays must be dealt with by the manager swiftly and decisively to reinforce the standard of ethical behavior.

Unintentional delay of care is an organizational systems issue. Such delays occur because of system failures, poorly designed systems, inadequate staff, or inappropriate facilities for accommodating a patient or patients. There are many chances for unintentional delays that should be monitored, such as the traffic within a busy emergency department or a busy high-risk unit where patients may not get the care they need on a timely basis. Such potential delays can cause considerable harm and must be addressed at the top of the organizational hierarchy (i.e., the parties responsible for providing appropriate systems, staff, equipment, and facilities). Failure to address such issues sends a negative message about the ethics of the organization.

Addressing and Ensuring an Ethical Culture

To establish and ensure an organizational culture based on ethics, several actions are necessary. These actions are addressed through a hierarchy of compliance. A hierarchical compliance model is shown in Figure 11-4.

As shown in the model, leadership with ethical values is the foundation of ethical compliance within the organization. Leadership starts with the CEO, the board, and the management team. Organizational policies outlining guidelines for ethical behavior are a must, followed with an assessment of the level of ethics within the organizational culture. Then, enforcement of compliance with ethical behavior guidelines is required as leadership holds themselves and the staff accountable for ethical conduct. The following paragraphs fully describe the levels of the model.

Leadership

There must be strong ethics evident at the top of the organization, starting with the CEO and including managers at all levels. The CEO must display a value set based on ethical and moral conduct, by "walking the talk" and providing an example for others. Lee Iacocca stated in his book, *Where Have All the Leaders Gone?*, "a leader has to be a person of character. That means knowing the difference between right and wrong and having the guts to do the right thing."[12] The CEO must hold everyone accountable for ethical behavior and, in turn, individual managers must do the same. To ensure an ethical team, the CEO has to recruit and retain a management team that reflects ethical values and holds their subordinates accountable for ethical behavior. Background and past conduct must be examined as part of the recruitment process, and job descriptions and performance evaluations must include compliance with ethics guidelines. The CEO must establish a code of ethics approved by the board; the duty of the CEO is to create a culture of ethics as job number one.

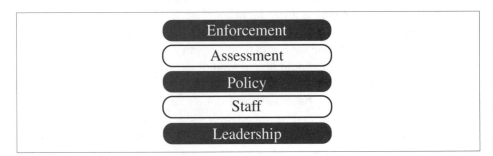

Figure 11-4 *Hierarchy of Compliance*

Governing Board

The governing board must establish and enforce standards of ethics for itself. The board must support the organization's leadership in establishing and enforcing an ethical culture. Karen Gardner states, in *The Excellent Board*, that selecting a qualified board with energy and passion to serve the community's most cherished institution is critical to the success of the healthcare organization.[13] Selection of board members with ethical values based on their history of behavior is critical to an ethical board and an ethical organization. The board must hold the CEO accountable for establishing standards of ethical conduct, and the board should require an annual evaluation that includes evaluation of the board's ethics as well as organization's ethics.

Staff

It is of utmost importance that the organization employs a staff of great people with strong ethical values. In *From Good to Great*, Collins provides strong evidence that some organizations are great because of the great people that make up the staff.[14] Great people are great because they have strong ethical values. It is well-known that one cannot teach a person ethics; one either does or does not possess ethics. It is that simple: Hire people with strong ethical values and teach them what they need to do the job. The reverse makes formation of an ethical culture impossible.

Ethics Policy

The organization must develop an ethics policy that addresses ethical behavior standards and describes how to identify and address ethical dilemmas and conflicts. The policy must address, for example, how to deal with gifts or with the monetary value limit if gifts are acceptable. The policy should include a definition of ethics and the principles and guidelines to follow when confronted with ethical conflicts and dilemmas. The ethics policy must be a part of orientation for all staff, be required at annual mandatory training sessions, and be reviewed during annual performance evaluations. Included in the policy should be a definition of descriptive and procedural justice along with disciplinary measures for unethical conduct. The policy also must provide mechanisms for addressing and reporting ethical conflicts. The policy should establish an ethics compliance hotline and hire an ethics officer to review ethical issues.

Ethics Consultant

To establish and to ensure ethical behavior, it is important to engage an ethics consultant to conduct an ethical assessment of leadership, the board, and the organization. The consultant can evaluate the state of ethics within the organization and provide recommendations to improve and ensure observance of ethical standards. The consultant can also inventory policies, procedures, and bylaws in the assessment of organizational justice, fairness, and compliance with ethical standards. The consultant can also conduct training for staff, managers, and board members.

Ethics Assessment and Evaluation

An annual ethics assessment and evaluation is recommended. This assessment should include a review of policies and procedures and compliance with their requirements. This activity should also include a review of ethical dilemmas and conflicts experienced during the year and note any observable trends in behavior. Lessons learned should be noted, including recommendations for preventing repetition of the same problems or errors. All employee evaluations should address ethics in the assessment of employee performance.

Enforcement

Leadership, including the CEO, the board, and the management team must enforce compliance with the established standards of ethical behavior as outlined in an organization's policies. It can also be helpful to establish an ethics hotline for employees to use to report apparent violations of ethical conduct and to voice their questions and concerns on matters of ethical behavior. Also, the organization may have its legal staff monitor ethical issues and recommended courses of actions to management.

Another suggestion for enforcing ethical standards involves conducting quarterly or semiannual case-study seminars for management and perhaps for the board. Case studies can be used to review what can be learned from publicized instances of unethical behavior involving well-known leaders and other national figures that appear to have violated reasonable ethical standards.

Andrew Kirtzman, in his book, *Betrayal: The Life and Lies of Bernie Madoff*, reports that Madoff had an epiphany at an early age when he realized that he could do everything he wanted if he simply lied to the people who trusted him the most.[15] Most leaders would agree that this revelation by Madoff is a chilling and disturbing motivation for getting ahead by taking advantage of the inborn instinct to trust. This book presents a classic example of how to evaluate the motives of leadership and how a purpose without ethics can destroy the morality of an individual and others and destroy the sanctity of trust.

Conclusion

Ethics is a complex subject that has been discussed, debated, and challenged throughout the centuries dating back to the ancient Greek and Roman era circa 400 BC. Today, ethics remains a major challenge for leaders and managers, especially in health care where people's lives must be embraced by a culture of ethics. The morality and trust in an organization are dependent on a strong foundation of ethics apparent from the top leadership down. The organization's leadership is entrusted and held accountable by the public to ensure a culture of ethics, morality, and trust. Ethics must be the guiding principle of the organization's mission and must be fully supported by all staff. Healthcare managers today must be constantly vigilant in knowing the boundaries of ethical and unethical behavior. They must also know that unethical behavior may also be illegal, such as hiring an unqualified friend or in taking bribes for personal gain.

Questions for Review and Discussion

1. Identify and describe two common areas of activity in which a manager may be tempted to be less than completely honest.
2. Describe what you believe to be the appropriate relationship between ethics and morality.
3. Why is an individual manager's visible ethical behavior important?
4. Identify and explain the strongest influences involved in ensuring an ethical culture.
5. Explain in detail why trust must be considered extremely fragile and how trust relates to confidence.
6. Describe in some detail the gray zone of the ethical continuum and some of the hazards that reside therein.
7. Describe how a culture of ethics is established and distributed throughout the organization.
8. In what ways is moral behavior shaped in the individual?
9. Name and describe the four unique ethical hazards faced by managers in healthcare organizations.
10. Why should the organization have a formal written ethics policy?

References

1. Lee, D. (Ed.). (trans. 1987). *Plato: The republic* (pp. xv–xvii). New York: Penguin Books.
2. Everitt, A. (2001). *Cicero: The life and times of Rome's greatest politician* (pp. vi–66). New York: Random House.
3. (1983). *The Holy Bible* (NKJV; Luke: 1–25). Nashville, TN: Thomas Nelson Publishers Cokesbury.
4. De Tocqueville, A. (1863/1984). *Democracy in America* (pp. 1–25). New York: Penguin Books.
5. Ethics. (1993). In *Merriam Webster's collegiate dictionary* (10th ed.; p. 398). Springfield, MA: Merriam-Webster, Inc.

6. Wood, A. W. (2001). *Basic writings of Kant* (p. vii). New York: The Modern Library.

7. Sayre-McCord, G. (Ed.). (2006). *David Hume: Moral philosophy* (pp. x–xxx, 361). Indianapolis, IN: Hackett Publishing Company.

8. Santrock, J. W. (2002). *Life-span development* (8th ed.; pp. 240–241). New York: McGraw-Hill.

9. Fukuyama, F. (1996). *Trust: The social virtues and the creation of prosperity* (p. 26). New York: Free Press.

10. Shore, D. (2005). *The trust prescription for healthcare: Building your reputation with consumers* (p. 4). Chicago, IL: Health Administration Press.

11. Covey, S. M. R. (2006). *The speed of trust: The one thing that changes everything* (pp. 1–5). New York: Free Press.

12. Iaccoca, L. (2007). *Where have all the leaders gone?* (p. 8). New York: Scriber.

13. Gardner, K. (2004). *The excellent board.* Chicago, IL: American Hospital Association Press.

14. Collins, J. (2001). *Good to great.* New York: Harper Collins Publishers.

15. Kirtzman, A. (2009). *Betrayal: The life and lies of Bernie Madoff.* New York: Harper Collins Publishers.

Chapter 12

Informed Consent and Patient Rights: Patient Self-Determination

Dawn M. Oetjen, PhD, *Program Director, MS, Health Services Administration, Department of Health Management and Informatics, College of Health & Public Affairs, University of Central Florida, Orlando, Florida*

Reid M. Oetjen, PhD, *Program Director, Executive MS, Health Services Administration, Department of Health Management and Informatics, College of Health & Public Affairs, University of Central Florida, Orlando, Florida*

Chapter Objectives

- Review the history and evolution of informed consent and convey its importance in the present-day provision of health care.
- Introduce and review the various elements and components of informed consent and the reasons for their existence.
- Review the types of informed consent and the rules and guidelines for determining who may provide consent.
- Address patient rights and responsibilities as set forth in the Patient Bill of Rights.
- Develop an understanding of the present-day uses of privacy and confidentiality and how these apply to individuals and to their personal medical information.

Informed Consent

Patients and their families are becoming increasingly more responsible as partners in their health care. One significant dimension of this expanded responsibility involves the use of informed consent.

As it is generally used, informed consent refers to both a legal document and the conditions addressed in that document. Recognized in all 50 states, informed consent conveys an individual's consent to a surgical or medical procedure or participation in a clinical study. It is based upon a clear appreciation and understanding of the facts, implications, and potential consequences of an action. The informed consent process is based on the moral and legal premise of patient autonomy, whereby patients have the right to make decisions about their health and medical conditions, and physicians have a duty to involve patients in decisions regarding their health care.

History

Informed consent, whether as a concept or the term itself, has often been traced back to the Nuremberg Trials during which 26 Nazi physicians were tried for research atrocities performed on prisoners of war and others. Resulting from these trials was the Nuremberg Code, the first recognized international code governing medical research. One of the primary foci of this chapter is to illuminate the requirement of *voluntary informed consent* of the human subject, thereby protecting the right of the individual to control his or her own body. This code also recognizes that risk must be weighed against the expected benefit, that unnecessary pain and suffering must be avoided, and that doctors should avoid actions that injure human patients.

The principles established by this code of medical practice have now been extended into general codes of medical ethics. Yet, as a code written in response to crimes against humanity, and, more specifically, written with regard to nontherapeutic human-subject research, the Nuremberg Code had little impact on the actual practice of therapeutic clinical research at the time of its writing, and, in fact, did not mention specifically informed consent.[1, 2]

More correctly, the term informed consent was believed by many to have been used first by Gebhard in a 1957 malpractice case, *Salgo v. Leland Stanford, Jr., the University Board of Trustees.*[3–5] In this case, the California Supreme Court stated that no patient can submit to a medical intervention without having given prior "informed consent." This ruling has been referenced for more than 45 years by medical historians, legal analysts, and medical ethicists as the event from which the term first originated.[2]

However, in 1995, the final report of the President's Advisory Committee on Human Radiation Experiments provided an even earlier history of the concept.[6] Through the committee's extensive research of archival materials from the Atomic Energy Commission (AEC), a letter was discovered, written in 1947 by the general manager of the newly formed AEC to a clinical investigator on an obscure and new requirement regarding the need for "informed consent." The letter was written specifically in response to the investigator's request to allow the declassification of data from government-sponsored radiation research on cancer patients, so that it might be reported and published by the investigator. As exemplified in the letter, the newly formed AEC clearly had significant concerns about potential litigation problems because of the use of seemingly vulnerable cancer patients as research subjects without any documentation of consent.[2]

Elements of Full Informed Consent

Although the specific definition of informed consent may vary from state to state, the elements of full informed consent are generally consistent. The physician must discuss with the individual involved the following elements:

- The individual's diagnosis (if known) and nature of the decision or proposed treatment or procedure;
- The benefits and risks of the decision or proposed treatment or procedure;
- Alternative decisions, treatments, or procedures;
- The benefits and risks of these alternatives;
- The benefits and risks of not receiving or undergoing any treatment or procedure;
- An opportunity for questions by individual and time for reflection;
- An assessment of patient understanding; and
- Acceptance (or refusal) of decision, treatment, procedure, or alternatives.

Components of Informed Consent

Informed consent involves more than simply getting a patient to sign a written consent form that outlines the aforementioned elements. It is a two-way communication process between an individual and physician that results in the individual's authorization or agreement to undergo a specific medical intervention.

There are four components of informed consent. First, in order to give informed consent, the individual concerned must have the capacity or ability to make the decision. Impairments to reasoning and judgment that would make it impossible to provide informed consent include conditions such as severe mental retardation, severe mental illness, intoxication, severe sleep deprivation, Alzheimer's disease, or being in a coma or persistent vegetative state (PVS).

Second, the individual must be in possession of all relevant facts at the time consent is given. There must be adequate disclosure of information. The law requires that a reasonable physician–patient standard be applied when determining how much information is considered adequate. There are three approaches to making this decision: (1) providing what the typical physician would say about the decision, treatment, or procedure (the reasonable physician standard); (2) providing what the average patient would say about the decision, treatment, or procedure (the reasonable patient standard); and (3) providing what this individual patient would need to know and understand to make an informed decision (the subjective standard).[7]

Third, the individual must comprehend the relevant information. The physician must evaluate whether or not the individual has understood what has been said, must ascertain that the risks have been accepted, and that the individual is giving consent to proceed with the decision, treatment, or procedure with full knowledge and forethought.[7] The individual shares this responsibility with the physician in that the physician may not realize that some items discussed were not understood until the individual asks questions or asks for more information.

And, fourth, individuals must voluntarily grant consent, without coercion or duress. Freedom of choice must exist, including the choice to go against medical advice and do nothing. To ensure that consent is voluntary, physicians should make clear to the individuals involved that they are actively participating in the decision and not simply signing a form.

Through addressing these four requirements, the following necessary conditions for informed consent are satisfied: (1) that the individual's decision is voluntary; (2) that the decision is made with an appropriate understanding of the circumstances; and (3) that the patient's choice is deliberate and that the patient has carefully considered all of the expected benefits, burdens, risks, and reasonable alternatives.

Types of Consent

Not all situations require that informed consent be given. For example, although listening to respirations through a stethoscope could be considered a treatment or procedure, it is not likely that a physician and patient would have a lengthy discussion about the risks and benefits of this care. This nonwritten consent that occurs when an individual cooperates with a particular action initiated by a physician is termed implied (indirect or deemed) consent.

Expressed (explicit or direct) consent, in oral or written form, should be obtained when the treatment or procedure is likely to be more than mildly painful or when it carries appreciable risk. If an individual were to agree to a surgical procedure, the physician would have the individual sign an expressed consent form.

Who Gives Consent?

Adults

Generally, adults, 18 years of age or older with decision-making capacity, are expected to make choices regarding their own treatment. Adults have decision-making capacity if they (1) have not been declared incompetent by the courts, and (2) are capable of evaluating alternatives, understanding the consequences of the alternatives, and selecting and acting accordingly. These decisions, made by competent adults, are usually outlined in advance directives, such as living wills. A surrogate decision maker or healthcare proxy may also be appointed by the individual to speak on their behalf. These advance directives and proxies are effective even if the individual becomes incapacitated.

If no advance directive exists and an individual is determined to be incapacitated or incompetent to make healthcare decisions, there is a specific hierarchy of appropriate decision makers defined by state law. In the absence of a state statute, the most widely accepted order of priority of close family is spouse, adult children, parents, adult siblings, and others. When there is more than one close family member or other person with knowledge of the individual's wishes, a family conference might be held to achieve consensus.[8] When consensus is not possible, or if there is no appropriate decision maker available, the physicians are expected to act in the best interest of the individual until a surrogate can be appointed. A court-appointed surrogate or proxy can also be appointed by a judge if requested by a physician, family member, friend, or an organization. This process varies from state to state.

Minors

If the individual is a minor, that is, younger than 18 years of age, the concept of informed consent has little direct application. Although minors may have appropriate decision-making capacity, they usually do not have the legal empowerment to give informed consent. Therefore, parents or other surrogate decision makers may give informed consent for diagnosis and treatment of a minor, preferably with the assent of the minor whenever possible. Most states also have laws that designate some minors as emancipated and entitled to the full rights of adults. These exceptions include minors who are: (1) self-supporting or not living in their parent's home; (2) married; (3) pregnant or a parent; (4) in the military; or (5) declared emancipated by a court. Most states also give decision-making authority to otherwise "mature minors" (unemancipated minors with decision-making capacity) who are seeking treatment for certain medical conditions, such as drug or alcohol abuse, pregnancy, or sexually transmitted diseases.[9]

No matter who is appointed to make the decision, the goal should remain the same: to make the decision that the individual would want if able to express it, and, if this is not known, to make the decision that is in the best interest of the individual.

When Consent Requirements Do Not Apply

An individual's consent should only be presumed, rather than obtained, in emergency situations when the individual is unconscious or incompetent and no surrogate decision maker is available. This privilege to proceed in emergency situations is extended to physicians because inaction at this time could cause greater harm to the patient and would be contrary to good medical practice; however, every effort should be made to document the urgent medical need for the procedure prior to proceeding.[10]

Managerial Implications

The process of obtaining informed consent, prevalent throughout healthcare facilities, is fraught with confusion, gaps, miscommunication, and potential for lawsuits. Most consent forms have been drafted by attorneys largely for attorneys and are difficult for many readers because of their complex legal terminology. In fact, researchers report that some 44% of patients who sign consent forms do not fully understand the exact nature of the procedure to be performed, and almost 70% did not read or understand the information on the form.[11]

Communicating the risks, benefits, and alternatives of procedures is often as challenging for the clinician as understanding is for the patient. Further complicating the matter is the fact that most physicians receive little or no training in how to communicate this information to their patients.[12] A prudent healthcare manager is advised to modify the informed consent process and offer one that is simplified yet complete, so there can be no doubt whether the patient has been informed.

For successful informed consent, there must be shared decision making such that patients are actively involved with their clinicians in reaching healthcare decisions. If this does not occur, interventions might be provided to patients who would not normally choose them and withheld from those who would.[13] Thus, it is critical that clinical personnel engage patients in a discussion about the nature and scope of the procedure and encourage patients to be active and informed participants in the process.[14] Healthcare organizations and clinicians are encouraged to make a commitment to transparency with patients about risks, benefits, and alternatives, whether good or bad.

One method of doing so involves creating forms that utilize simple language, translated as necessary into the primary language of the patient. This sort of consent form should be used as a guide for the essential discussion between physician and patient. The National Quality Forum (NQF) suggests that healthcare organizations then ask patients or their surrogates to repeat what has been told to them in their own words to ensure that the elements of the informed consent discussion are understood.

When working with patients exhibiting weak proficiency in English, a low literacy level, or problems with vision or hearing, appropriate accommodations should be made.[14] Healthcare organizations should provide patients with the necessary assistance; the costs of doing so are inconsequential when considered relative to the legal implications of failing to do so. Additionally, clinicians need to be sensitive to patients' cultural beliefs and practices in order to avoid misunderstandings.

Patients' Rights and Responsibilities

In addition to informed consent, there are numerous other patient rights and responsibilities. These are articulated in the *Consumer Bill of Rights and Responsibilities* that was adopted by the US Advisory Commission on Consumer Protection and

Quality in the Health Care Industry in 1988. It is also known as the *Patient Bill of Rights* and was created with the intent of reaching three major goals: (1) to help patients feel more confident in the US healthcare system by ensuring that the system is fair and that it works to meet patients' needs, gives patients a way to address any problems they may have, and encourages patients to take an active role in staying or getting healthy; (2) to stress the importance of a strong relationship between patients and their healthcare providers; and (3) to stress the key role patients play in staying healthy by laying out rights and responsibilities for all patients and healthcare providers. These rights and responsibilities include: information disclosure, choice of providers and plans, access to emergency services, participation in treatment decisions, respect and nondiscrimination, privacy and confidentiality of health information, and complaints and appeals.[15]

Information Disclosure

In addition to being well-informed about the treatment options available to them, individuals have the right to accurately and easily understand information about their health plans along with the healthcare professionals and facilities that are available to choose from or those who are already their care providers. Information regarding health care can be quite complex and often cannot be explained to or understood by an individual at any literacy level. Whenever possible, this information should be clearly and concisely written in a manner that can be understood by all, or at a maximum, a 4th grade level of reading. While the average literacy level of Americans is typically higher (at about a 7th or 8th grade reading level), the terminology used in health care is more complex and intimidating to readers; therefore, writing at a lower level is less likely to hinder comprehension.

Additionally, the United States is a melting pot of many cultures, each with its own language and customs. Facilities should ensure that individuals receive from all staff members effective, understandable, and respectful care that is provided in a manner compatible with cultural health beliefs and practices and in the individual's preferred language. Language assistance services, including bilingual staff and interpreter services, should be offered at no cost to individuals with limited English proficiency at all points of contact in a timely manner and during all hours of operation. Facilities should also make available easily understood health-related materials and post signage in the languages of the commonly encountered groups and/or groups represented in the service area.[16]

Choice of Providers and Plans

With the continually rising cost of health care and the frequently encountered barriers to accessing care, individuals deserve the opportunity to exercise choice regarding treatment providers and options. The concept of choice is deeply ingrained in American consumers and can be traced back to the guarantees provided in the

US Constitution. Thus, individuals should have both the expectation and the right to personally choose properly trained and credentialed healthcare providers who can furnish high quality health care when it is needed. This right to choose one's own healthcare facilities, providers, and health plans is considered sacred by many, and any threat can quickly mobilize consumers to fight to retain their right.

Access to Emergency Services

Individuals have the right to access emergency healthcare services when and where the need arises. Health plans use a "prudent layperson" standard in determining eligibility for coverage of emergency services. Coverage of emergency department services must be available without authorization if there is reason to believe an individual's life is in danger or that the person would be seriously injured or disabled without immediate care. Individuals have the right to be screened and stabilized using emergency services and should be able to use these services whenever and wherever needed, without having to wait for authorization and without financial penalty.

Participation in Treatment Decisions

As discussed in the previous section, individuals have the right to know their treatment options and to take part in decisions about their care. For persons who may be incompetent or unable to make these decisions, parents, guardians, family members, or others selected by the individual can represent them.

Additionally, individuals have the right to refuse treatment. Except for legally authorized involuntary treatment, persons who are legally competent to make medical decisions and who are judged by healthcare providers to have decision-making capacity have the legal and moral right to refuse any and all treatment. This is true even if the individual chooses to use poor judgment that may result in serious disability or even death.

Individuals also have the right to refuse information or to ask that only minimal information be given to them and, instead, rely on the health provider to make decisions regarding their care. The healthcare provider should make sure that the individual has clearly expressed this refusal in writing.

Respect and Nondiscrimination

Individuals have a right to considerate, nondiscriminatory, and respectful care from healthcare providers and health plan representatives at all times and under all circumstances. Individuals must not be discriminated against in the delivery of healthcare services, consistent with the benefits covered in their policy or as required by law. Individuals who are eligible for coverage under the terms and conditions of a health plan or program or as required by law also must not be discriminated against in marketing and enrollment practices based on race, ethnicity, national origin, religion, sex, age, mental or physical disability, sexual orientation, genetic information, or source of payment. This environment of mutual respect is essential to maintaining a quality healthcare system.[15]

Privacy and Confidentiality of Health Information

The Health Insurance Portability and Accountability Act (HIPAA) Privacy Rule provides federal guidelines to protect the confidentiality of identifiable medical information (see Chapter 2). It also gives individuals more control over and knowledge regarding the persons or entities who will be using their medical information and for what purposes. Also, the HIPAA Patient Safety Rule protects identifiable information from being used to analyze patient safety events and improve patient safety (see Chapter 2 for additional information concerning HIPAA).

Privacy

Privacy and confidentiality are terms that are often used interchangeably; however, in actuality, they are largely separate concepts. Privacy is an individual's right to control the access of oneself by others. Individuals decide with whom, when, and where to share their personal information. For example, individuals may not want to be seen entering places that might stigmatize them, or they may not want to share certain diagnoses with their employers.

To ensure that an individual's privacy is not breached, there are certain measures that can be taken by healthcare organizations. These measures include the following: (1) Discussions and consultations containing identifiable patient information should take place in areas that afford discretion and confidentiality, and never in elevators, hallways, cafeterias, or other areas where nonmedical staff may be present. (2) Common courtesies, such as knocking on doors before entering and closing bedside curtains prior to initiating physical exams should be extended to all individuals. (3) Discretion should be observed when leaving messages on answering machines or when faxing information. (4) Individuals should be informed of all personnel present and involved in their care, including observers, interns, and medical students.

Confidentiality

Privacy generally concerns people, whether singly or in concert. Confidentiality, however, concerns information. Today's enlightened outlook concerning confidentiality conveys the belief that information about an individual should be controllable by that individual, and that the individual has the right to specify what personal information can be communicated and to whom it can be communicated. Thus, policies concerning information handling are placed before all who enter the health-care system, and individuals must designate who, if anyone other than the providers involved in their care, is entitled to access to that information.

Privacy and confidentiality certainly overlap to some extent, especially in situations in which breaching confidentiality may also entail invading privacy. Consider the simplest of examples: You are hospitalized in a unit that is identified with a particular kind of medical problem. You want no one to know where you are and you want no one to visit you. But someone "slips" and advises an intended visitor where you are; the room and unit identification set you up for a violation of privacy because others now know where you are, and a breach of confidentiality has occurred because one can infer from the information received what your medical issue might be as well as knowing you are indeed hospitalized. Thus, privacy and confidentiality, though separable concepts, are frequently found hand-in-hand.

Complaints and Appeals

You have the right to a fair, fast, and objective review of any complaint you have against your health plan, hospitals, doctors, or other healthcare personnel. This includes complaints about waiting times, hours of operation, the actions of healthcare personnel, and the adequacy of healthcare facilities.

In a healthcare system that protects consumers' rights, it is reasonable to expect and to encourage consumers to assume reasonable responsibilities. Greater individual involvement by consumers in their care increases the likelihood of achieving the best outcomes and helps support a quality improvement and, cost-conscious environment.

The individual as a consumer can make a significant contribution in several key areas, such as by:

- Maximizing healthy habits (e.g., exercising, not smoking, and following a healthy diet);
- Becoming involved in care decisions;
- Working collaboratively with providers in developing and carrying out agreed-upon treatment plans;
- Disclosing relevant information and clearly communicating wants and needs;
- Using available disputed-claims processes when there is disagreement between individual and health plan (the process is described in plan brochures);
- Becoming knowledgeable of coverage and health plan options, including covered benefits, limitations and exclusions, rules regarding use of network providers, coverage and referral rules, appropriate processes to secure additional information, and process to appeal coverage decisions (this information is in plan brochures);
- Showing respect for other patients and for healthcare workers;
- Making a good-faith effort to meet financial obligations; and
- Reporting wrongdoing and fraud to appropriate resources or legal authorities.

Questions for Review and Discussion

1. In what ways have people not always had complete control over their own health care?

2. What do you believe is the "moral and legal premise of patient autonomy?"

3. In what ways are the patients of today being encouraged to take more responsibility for their own care?

4. Who may automatically access your personal health information without your signed permission?

5. It is understood that in its use in this chapter, consent means the granting of permission to deliver some form of care to the individual, but what makes it *informed* consent?

6. Explain in your own words the objectives of the Patient Bill of Rights.

7. What courses of action are available if an individual does not or is in no position to grant consent for medical care?

8. What is the primary purpose of an advance directive?

9. Explain in detail the differences between an advance directive and a health-care proxy.

10. What are the requirements that must be fulfilled for informed consent to be legal and valid?

References

1. Faden, R. R., Beauchamp, T. L., & King, N. M. P. (1986). *A history and theory of informed consent.* New York, NY: Oxford University Press.

2. Daugherty, C. K. (1999, May). Impact of therapeutic research on informed consent and the ethics of clinical trials: A medical oncology perspective. *Journal of Clinical Oncology, 17*(5), 1601.

3. Salgo v. Leland Stanford, Jr., the University Board of Trustees, 317 P 2nd 170 (1957).

4. Katz, J. (1984). *The silent world of doctor and patient.* New York: The Free Press.

5. P. G. Gebhard, 69, developer of the term "informed consent" [obituary]. (1997, August 26). *The New York Times.*

6. Advisory Committee on Human Radiation Experiments. (1996). *The human radiation experiments* (pp. 46–67). New York: Oxford University Press.

7. Informed consent. (Eds.). (2005). In J. Lehman & S. Phelps (Eds.), *West's encyclopedia of American law.* Detroit: Thomson Gale.

8. Miller, R. D. (2006). *Problems in health care law.* Sudbury, MA: Jones and Bartlett Publishers.

9. American Academy of Pediatrics, Committee on Bioethics. (1995, February). Informed consent, parental permission, and assent in pediatric practice. *Pediatrics, 95*(2), 314–317.

10. Pozgar, G. (2010). *Legal and ethical issues for health professionals.* Sudbury, MA: Jones and Bartlett Publishers.

11. National Quality Forum. (2005). *Implementing a national voluntary consensus standard for informed consent. A user's guide for healthcare professionals*. Washington, DC: Author. Available at: http://www.qualityforum.org/Publications/2005/09/Implementing_a_National_Voluntary_Consensus_Standard_for_Informed_Consent__A_User%E2%80%99s_Guide_for_Healthcare_Professionals.aspx. Accessed June 29, 2010.

12. Schwartz, L. M., Woloshin, S., & Welch, H. G. (1999). Risk communication in clinical practice: Putting cancer into context. *Journal of the National Cancer Institute, 1999*(25), 124–133.

13. Sepucha, K. R., Fowler, F. J., & Mulley, A. G. (2004, October 7). Policy support for patient-centered care: The need for measurable improvements in decision quality. *Health Affairs*.

14. The Joint Commission. (2009). *Patient safety essentials for health care* (5th ed.). Oak Brook Terrace, IL: Joint Commission Resources.

15. President's Advisory Commission on Consumer protection and Quality in the Health Care Industry. (1998). *Consumer Bill of Rights and Responsibilities*. Available at: http://govinfo.library.unt.edu/hcquality/cborr. Accessed November 23, 2009.

16. The Office of Minority Health. (2007*). National Standards on Culturally and Linguistically Appropriate Services (CLAS)*. Available at: http://minorityhealth.hhs.gov/templates/browse.aspx?lvl=2&lvlID=15. Accessed November 17, 2009.

Chapter 13

Legal Aspects of Nursing: Protecting Your Patients and Your License

Tejal Banker, JD, LLM, *Healthcare Attorney and Adjunct Faculty, Healthcare Administration, University of Houston-Clear Lake, Houston, Texas*

Ashish Chandra, MBA, PhD, *Professor and Department Chair, Healthcare Administration, University of Houston-Clear Lake, Houston, Texas*

Chapter Objectives

- Identify and define the various causes of action that have the potential for involving a nurse in a negligence or medical malpractice lawsuit either individually or as an employee of a provider organization.
- Develop an appreciation of the hazards and potential consequences of involvement in a malpractice action.
- Review the various sources of law applicable to a medical malpractice or negligence situation.
- Overview the various stages of a medical malpractice lawsuit.
- Provide information and guidance for nurses and nurse managers to apply in avoiding malpractice charges.

Introduction

Recent decades have seen a steady increase in the number of lawsuits filed against nurses. Many nurses are employees of individual healthcare providers such as physicians or healthcare facilities such as hospitals or nursing homes. Healthcare providers are typically held liable for the negligent acts of their employees if such acts are within the scope of the employees' duties. However, a nurse's status as an employee will not always immunize him or her against being held liable for medical negligence. Thus a nurse who is an employee of a healthcare provider can be named as a defendant in a medical malpractice lawsuit. Furthermore, if a healthcare provider is held liable for the negligent act of its nurse employee, such healthcare providers can seek monetary indemnification from the nurse employee.

Many causes of action can be brought against a nurse. Most lawsuits filed against nurses involve allegations of medical negligence, that is, medical malpractice. Although, in many instances, only the physician or the hospital is named as a defendant in a medical malpractice lawsuit, increasingly, nurses are also being named, or at least being subpoenaed to appear as witnesses. More than ever, today's nurses are increasingly exposed to lawsuits because of increases in:

- The occurrence of mistakes due to: (1) increased autonomy and a greater-than-ever scope of responsibility, (2) higher levels of standards of care, and (3) fatigue caused by increase in patient loads and staffing shortages;
- Patient expectations for favorable outcomes due to advances in medical technology;[1]
- A dependence on technology to capture and convey medical information, and the use of nurse-assistive personnel to provide healthcare services;[1] and
- The litigious nature of society.[2]

The expanding role of the nurse in our healthcare system is surely capable of decreasing the costs of providing health care; however, medical negligence attributable to nursing errors can ultimately lead to increased costs. Just as any other healthcare professional, a nurse can be held accountable for unintentional and intentional acts that harm a patient. Because of the increasing rate at which nurses are being named as defendants in medical negligence lawsuits, it is imperative that every nurse develop a basic understanding of the legal aspects of nursing by becoming thoroughly familiar with:

- The sources of nursing law;
- The anatomy of a lawsuit;
- The causes of action that can be asserted against a nurse;
- The theories of liability; and
- The measures that can be taken to avoid a lawsuit.

The Sources of Nursing Law

Familiarization with the various sources of law forms the basis for understanding the legal aspects of nursing. Law can be classified as either public law or private law.[3] Public law regulates the interaction between the government and its citizens and businesses. Private law regulates the conduct, rights, and duties among individuals.

There are four main sources of law in the United States: written constitutions, judicial decisions, statutes, and administrative law.

The US Constitution is the quintessential example of a written constitution. The US Constitution is the supreme law of the land. The US Constitution provides the framework for the organization of the government and for organizing the relationship of the federal government to the states, to citizens, and to all people within the United States; defines the powers of each branch of the government; and reserves all unenumerated powers to the states and to the people. Each state has its own constitution which is subordinate to the federal constitution.

The judicial decision is a second major source of law. The judicial branch of the government is responsible for the adjudication of disputes based on the parties involved in any particular lawsuit and the specific issues that are raised by that lawsuit. Judicial decisions are the primary source of private law. Private law, specifically, the law of contracts and torts, has traditionally had the most influence on health care.[3] The role of the courts is to interpret statutes or regulations. In rendering their decisions, courts are bound by the principle of *stare decisis*. Stare decisis requires that courts look to past disputes involving similar facts to determine the outcome of the case at issue. The use of earlier court cases as precedent certainly contributes to stability in the legal system; however, precedent is not absolute and a court in a jurisdiction outside that of the initial trial court can render a different decision.

The third source of law is statutes. Statutes help to maintain a government's right to protect individual rights[3] and are enacted by federal or state legislators or a unit of local government.[3] The role of the judiciary is to interpret statutes. The nurse practice acts of the fifty states and the District of Columbia are examples of statutes. The nurse practice act of each state sets the standards for the nursing profession in that state and outlines the activities a licensed nurse may perform. Although one state's nurse practice act will differ from that of another state, the following elements are common to all nurse practice acts:

- A definition of professional nursing;
- Requirements for licensure and possible exemptions from state licensure laws;
- Requirements for relicensure;
- Means for disciplinary action and requirements for due process concerning violations of the nurse practice act, including private reprimand or warning, public reprimand, probation, suspension of license, refusal to renew license, and license revocation;
- Criteria for creating the state board of nursing and for designating members to service on the board; and
- Penalties for practicing without a license.[4]

Administrative law is a fourth source of law. Administrative agencies are given power by the legislature to operate within their specific enumerated areas. Administrative agencies have the authority to create rules and regulations that take on the force of statute. A state board of nursing is an example of an administrative agency. Because a state's legislature has neither the time nor the specialized knowledge to enforce a state's nurse practice act, a key role of a state's nursing board is to draft implementing regulations for the state's nurse practice act and to enforce that state's nurse practice act. The board of nursing of any state also serves the following functions:

- Proposing revisions to the state's nurse practice act;
- Supervising the licensing of individual nurses;
- Establishing and monitoring adherence with continuing education requirements; and
- Reprimanding, suspending, or revoking the licenses of individual nurses.

The Anatomy of a Lawsuit

Being named as nurse defendant in a medical malpractice lawsuit can be emotionally draining for the nurse and financially detrimental to the nurse's employer. There may also be financial implications for any nurse who is found to have been acting beyond the scope of his or her employment. Lawsuits are time consuming, and, regardless of the outcome, most any lawsuit can generate negative publicity. However, familiarity with the legal process can improve predictability in a challenging situation.

The First Stage

The first stage of a lawsuit involves filing a legal action. A claimant who files a lawsuit is the plaintiff, and the other party is the defendant. The lawsuit begins when the plaintiff files a complaint stating the charges against the defendant and identifying the damages sought. In a medical malpractice case, a patient will often name the hospital, the attending physicians, and attending nurses as defendants, and will identify economic damages sought, such as compensation for lost wages and medical expenses. There may also be compensation sought for noneconomic damages, such as pain and suffering and emotional distress. A copy of the complaint, along with a summons enumerating the plaintiff's charges, is then served on the defendant.

The Second Stage

In the second stage of a lawsuit, once the defendant is served with the summons and complaint, the defendant files an answer to the complaint in which the defendant admits, denies, or pleads ignorance to each allegation. The defendant's answer may also ask the court to dismiss the complaint. If the court grants the defendant's motion to dismiss, the judgment becomes final. The plaintiff has the option to appeal the decision. The defendant may also add a counterclaim to the plaintiff's charges.

The Third Stage

Discovery is the third stage of a lawsuit. Discovery is a process through which both plaintiff and defendant gather information and assess the strength of the other party's position. Depositions, interrogatories, demands to inspect and copy documents, demands for physical or mental examination of a party, and requests for admission of facts are five methods that may be employed to ascertain the strength of the opposing party's case.

Interrogatories are written questions that must be answered in writing. Physical and mental examinations are discovery methods that may be utilized when the physical or mental condition of a party in the lawsuit is in dispute. Depositions and demands to inspect and copy documents are discovery devices that are utilized in medical malpractice cases as well as in certain other lawsuits. During each deposition, a witness testifies under oath before a court reporter who transcribes the testimony. In medical malpractice cases, both plaintiff and defendant often depose expert witnesses who assess the facts and circumstances, and provide their opinions as to the requisite standard of care.

When a nurse is a defendant, the best expert witness for the defense is another nurse with a similar level of experience and education. Demands to inspect and copy documents are discovery methods whereby a party inspects and copies items in the other party's possession such as books, specific documents, personnel files, and other business records, and, in medical malpractice cases, patient medical records.

The Fourth and Fifth Stages

During the fourth and fifth stages of the lawsuit, the court hears statements from both plaintiff and defendant. The court attempts to narrow and clarify the issues, and either or both parties may attempt negotiation or may present offers in an effort to settle the case outside of court. Often, in an effort to contain costs and obtain a swift resolution, the parties will try to reach an out-of-court settlement. If the parties are unable to reach a resolution, the case will go to trial.

The Sixth Stage

The actual trial is the sixth stage of the lawsuit. It commences with the selection of a jury if either the plaintiff or defendant has requested a jury trial. After the jury is selected, the attorney for the plaintiff and the attorney for the defendant each give opening statements in which they present the facts as they apply to their respective cases. After the opening statements, the plaintiff presents its case by calling witnesses and presenting other evidence. In a nursing malpractice case, a plaintiff's attorney may call a nurse as an expert witness to testify and provide opinions regarding specific aspects of the case. While the plaintiff's side is presenting its case, the defense attorney is given the opportunity to question the plaintiff's witnesses.

After the plaintiff's case is presented, the defense attorney may ask the court to direct a verdict for the defense. If the motion is denied, the defendant's case will be presented by producing witnesses and evidence. While the defendant's case is being presented, the plaintiff's attorney is given the opportunity to question the defense's witnesses.

After the defense closes its case, each side summarizes its position in closing statements and either party may move for a directed verdict. If the court denies the motions, the judge will instruct the jury regarding the relevant law, and the jury will review the facts and deliberate until it reaches a verdict. The jury then announces the verdict to the court.

Either party may appeal the judgment. The appellate court will limit itself to a review of the applicable law and will not relitigate the facts. The appellate court may affirm the decision of the lower court, modify or reverse the decision, or reverse the decision and remand the case for a new trial.

Causes of Action

Causes of action brought against nurses commonly fall under the purview of tort law.[4] The law of torts addresses injuries by one party against another party for which the injured party may sue the alleged wrongdoer for damages. The two types of torts are intentional torts and unintentional torts.[4] All intentional torts include the following elements:

- The intention to interfere with the plaintiff or the plaintiff's property;
- The intention to bring about the consequences of the act; and
- The act is a substantial factor in bringing about the consequences.[4]

Assault, battery, false imprisonment, and intentional infliction of emotional distress are all examples of intentional torts with which nurses could be charged.[4] A nurse found guilty of assault, battery, false imprisonment, or intentional infliction of emotional distress could be held both criminally and civilly liable.

An unintentional tort is an unintended, yet wrongful act that causes harm to another person.[4] Negligence is a type of unintentional tort under which a wrongdoer is generally held to be civilly liable (as opposed to criminally liable). Medical negligence, also known as medical malpractice, is the most common cause of action brought against nurses. Medical malpractice can be defined as negligence on the part of a healthcare practitioner, such as a physician or nurse, which causes physical or emotional damage to a patient to whom a duty of care is owed.

Assault is a type of intentional tort that a nurse could be charged with. Assault is a wrongful, intentional act by one person that creates apprehension in another of an immediate harmful or offensive contact.[5] The action can be an apparent attempt to inflict harm, such as raising a fist in a threatening manner. A key element in proving an assault cause of action is apprehension of being touched; no actual physical contact needs to occur.[5] A verbal threat to touch another in an injurious or offensive manner could be considered an assault if the other party felt that he or she was in imminent danger of harm.[5]

Battery is the most common intentional tort that is asserted against nurses.

Battery is the intentional harmful or offensive physical contact with another person without that person's consent.[4] The following elements must be proven to establish a case for battery:

- An act done by an individual;
- An intent to cause harmful or offensive contact on the part of said individual; and
- Harmful or offensive contact with another.[6]

The victim need not have any apprehension of imminent harm for the act to be deemed a battery.[4] It is important to note that a victim does not have to be touched personally in order to bring about a battery cause of action against the alleged wrongdoer. If a patient is harmed, even accidently, by an object in the hands of a nurse, or by an object that is set in motion by any action of a nurse, that nurse may be liable for battery.[5] Treatment without consent of a patient is the most commonly alleged act of battery involving nurses.[5]

False imprisonment is the intentional, illegal detention of a person without his or her consent and without valid justification for the confinement.[5] A nurse can be accused of false imprisonment when he or she uses physical restraints or confines a patient without legal justification for doing so.[4] Nurses must prove that, in their professional opinion, there was valid reason for the physical restraints or the seclusion of the individual, and a nurse who is unable to substantiate the action risks a charge of false imprisonment.

Intentional *infliction of emotional distress* is another type of intentional tort that can be brought against a nurse. The following elements must be satisfied in order to establish a case of intentional infliction of emotional distress:

- The alleged wrongdoer must act intentionally or recklessly;
- The nurse's conduct must be extreme and outrageous; and
- The nurse's conduct must be the cause of severe emotional distress.[5]

A nurse charged with assault, battery, or false imprisonment can also be charged with intentional infliction of emotional distress.

Negligence is an unintentional tort; it is the most common cause of action asserted against healthcare practitioners for medical errors. In the nursing context, negligence (or malpractice) is the failure of a nurse to act as a reasonable and prudent nurse would have acted in the same or similar circumstances. To prove liability on the part of a nurse, a patient must prove the following elements:

- The nurse owed him or her a duty to care;
- The nurse breached the standard of care;
- The patient suffered injury; and
- The nurse's breach of duty was both the legal and factual cause of the patient's injury.

A negligence cause of action against a nurse can exist only if the nurse owes a duty to a patient. A nurse has a duty to care for a patient once he or she accepts report and is assigned a patient. By accepting an assigned patient, the nurse acquires a duty to care for the patient with the degree of skill and prudence that would be exercised by a similarly situated nurse.

The second element of a malpractice cause of action against a nurse involves establishing the standard of care at the time the alleged malpractice occurred and proving that the nurse violated the standard of care. The standard of care is defined as the level of care that would be exercised by an ordinary, reasonable, and prudent healthcare practitioner in similar circumstances. The following can be used to establish the standard of care:

- Hospital policies and procedures;
- A state's nurse practice act;
- Guidelines, policies, and procedures for nursing care delivery published by national nursing organizations, state boards of nursing, credentialing bodies, and the Joint Commission;
- Nursing care plans;
- Published court opinions;
- Administrative codes such as the Patient Bill of Rights and manuals published by the Centers for Medicare and Medicaid Services; and
- Nursing texts and journals.[8]

Expert testimony is often utilized in medical malpractice cases to establish the standard of care and to determine whether a breach of the standard of care occurred. The plaintiff's expert will try to establish that the nurse breached the standard of care and the nurse's expert will try to establish that the nurse acted in accordance with the standard of care. An expert in a nursing malpractice case is usually a nurse who has a similar level of experience as the defendant, who specializes in the defendant's area of practice, and who is not otherwise involved in the case.[4]

Once the appropriate standard of care is established, the plaintiff must establish that the nurse violated the standard. A breach of the standard of care may be said to occur if the nurse fails to exercise the degree of care that a reasonable nurse would have exercised in similar circumstances. Examples of breach in the standard of care include:

- Failure to adhere to the nurse practice act of the state in which the nurse is licensed;
- Failure to follow the standard of care;
- Failure to adhere to policy, protocol, or procedure;
- Failure to document;
- Failure to recognize change in patient condition;

- Failure to appreciate a change in patient condition;
- Failure to follow up a change in patient condition;
- Failure to communicate within the healthcare hierarchy;
- Failure to monitor;
- Failure to act as patient advocate; and
- Failure to provide a safe environment.[2]

Once a plaintiff establishes that a nurse breached the accepted standard of care, the plaintiff must then establish that such a breach was both a factual and legal cause of the patient's injury. Even if the nurse deviated from the usual standard of care, the nurse will not be deemed negligent if, in fact, such deviation was not both the factual and legal cause of the patient's injury. For example, failing to properly document treatment rendered to a patient certainly deviates from the standard of care; however, a nurse could not be deemed negligent if such failure to document did not cause injury or did not cause the injury at issue. In order to establish factual causation, the patient must prove that his or her injury would not have occurred but for the nurse's breach of the standard of care. A determination of legal causation rests on the remoteness of a patient's harm from the negligence of a nurse. A nurse's negligence will be considered too remote, and therefore not a legal cause, if it is determined that a reasonable person could not foresee such injury occurring from such negligence.[4]

Finally, a negligence cause of action requires the plaintiff to incur damages. The plaintiff's attorney must prove that the nurse's breach resulted in injury to a patient. A patient can recover both economic and noneconomic damages in a negligence lawsuit. Economic damages are damages that can be monetarily quantified. Examples of economic damages include loss of earnings and past and future medical expenses. Noneconomic damages are damages for intangible harm, such as pain, emotional distress, disfigurement, loss of enjoyment of life, and loss of a loved one. Noneconomic damages are not easy to quantify with a dollar amount. In an effort to reduce the frequency of medical malpractice lawsuits, some states have statutorily imposed limits on a plaintiff's recovery for noneconomic damages. Texas, for example, generally limits a patient's recovery for noneconomic damages to $250,000.

The doctrine of *respondeat superior*, which means "let the master answer" forms the basis of liability in many nursing negligence cases. Under the doctrine of respondeat superior, an employer is liable for the negligent act of its employee if such act took place during the term of employment and if the employee was acting within the scope of employment when such act took place. The rationale for the respondeat superior theory of liability is that the employer benefits from the actions of its employee and so the employer should be held liable for the negligent actions of its employee occurring within the scope of such employee's employment. An employee's conduct will be considered to be within the scope of employment if it is of the nature that the individual is employed to perform and is, at least in part, in furtherance of his or her duties to the employer. Under the doctrine of respondeat superior, a healthcare institution such as a hospital can be held liable for the negligent acts of its nurse employees. If the hospital is found liable under the theory of respondeat superior, the hospital will have to pay all legal costs of defending the suit even if the hospital is not named as a defendant. However, if the nurse employee's negligent act arose out of actions that were not within the scope of the nursing practice, the health-care institution will not be held liable. Accordingly, a hospital that is named as a defendant in a nursing negligence lawsuit will try to prove that the nurse's negligence arose out of actions that were outside the scope of his or her employment. Whenever a nurse employee acts outside of the scope of his or her employment by, for example, performing duties that are reserved for a physician or a nurse practitioner, he or she risks of being held personally liable in a medical malpractice suit and, consequently, bearing the entire burden of defending a medical malpractice lawsuit.

Special applications of the doctrine of respondeat superior applicable in the medical malpractice context are the "borrowed servant" and "captain-of-the-ship" doctrines. Under the borrowed servant and captain-of-the-ship doctrines, a nurse employed by a healthcare institution such as a hospital is a temporary servant of a physician for the duration of that physician's surgical case. The physician supervises the conduct of the nurse and has assumed control of all of the medical personnel and events that take place in the surgical suite. Accordingly, if a nurse committed a negligent act while he or she was "loaned" to the physician, the physician (as opposed to the hospital) could then be held liable for the nurse's negligence.

What to Do to Avoid a Lawsuit

A nurse's involvement in a medical lawsuit brought by a patient can be professionally devastating in the following ways:

- The employer will likely terminate the nurse's employment if the nurse is found guilty of malpractice;
- A nurse will likely be required to report involvement in malpractice suits to each future employer;
- State nursing boards are likely to suspend or discipline nurses who are found guilty in medical malpractice law suits; and
- Any adverse action taken against a nurse will be reported to insurers and the National Practitioners Data Bank.

Nurses should be familiar with the procedural aspects of the legal process and the causes of action that can be asserted. However, every nurse should also be cognizant of the steps that can be taken to avoid being named as a defendant in a lawsuit by a patient or, if actually named as a defendant, be familiar with the ways in which liability can be negated.

Familiarity with and adherence to the rules and regulations embodied in the applicable state nurse practice act, healthcare provider policies and procedures, and nursing society policies and procedures provides a principal means of avoiding nursing errors. A state's nurse practice act defines the scope of a nurse's duties and serves as the standard by which a nurse's behavior is judged. In medical negligence cases in which a nurse is named as a defendant, the standard of care is established by the applicable state's nurse practice act, the employer's policies and procedures, and the policy and procedures of the appropriate nursing society. If a nurse acts in compliance with the nurse practice act and all employer and professional rules, the nurse will be relieved of liability.

Another way for a nurse to avoid involvement in a medical malpractice lawsuit is to adhere to the established scope of his or her practice. Nurses are sometimes delegated tasks that they are not qualified to perform; however, performance of such tasks is to be avoided. It may not be easy to decline, even as diplomatically as possible, the performance of a task that lies outside of one's legal ability to perform, but it is ultimately much safer to decline to perform such a task, while stating the reason for doing so, than it is to step outside of one's legitimate scope of practice. By providing care that is within the scope of a nurse's practice, a nurse reduces the personal risk of error and, thus, reduces the risk of liability.

Correct, detailed documentation is another means that may relieve a nurse of liability if he or she is named as a defendant in a lawsuit. Charting is integral to proving that the nurse met the applicable standard of care. Without proper documentation, it becomes extremely difficult to prove that the nurse acted in accordance with the applicable standard of care.

Questions for Review and Discussion

1. What is your understanding of the borrowed servant doctrine? Explain how this doctrine can potentially affect a nurse's position in a legal action.
2. When might a healthcare employer not be liable for the actions of an employed nurse?
3. What are the sources of administrative law as applicable to nurses?
4. Thoroughly explain the importance of documentation in a healthcare organization's defense of a lawsuit.
5. Why does assault not necessarily have to involve actual physical contact?
6. Describe what an unintentional tort is and offer examples for discussion.
7. Why can a healthcare organization be held responsible for the actions of its employees?
8. It has been claimed that the tendency for patients to initiate lawsuits has increased in recent years. Why might this be so?

9. Describe a situation in which a nurse could potentially be charged with false imprisonment.

10. How might a healthcare organization go about defending its standards of care?

References

1. Shinn, L. J. (2001). *Yes you can be sued*. The Nursing Risk Management Series. Available at: https://nursingworld.org/mods/archive/mod310/cerm101.htm. Accessed June 29, 2010.

2. sirI. (2008, July 4). *Litigious areas of nursing and the nurse's liability* [Web log post]. Available at: http://allnurses.com/nursing-blogs/litigious-areas-nursing-337239.html. Accessed June 29, 2010.

3. Showalter, S. J. (2007). The law of healthcare administration (5th ed., pp. 1–22). Chicago: Health Administration Press.

4. Catalano, J. T. (1994). *Ethical and legal aspects of nursing* (2nd ed.). Springhouse, PA: Springhouse Corporation.

5. Sharpe, C. (1999). *Nursing malpractice: Liability and risk management*. Westport, CT: Greenwood Publishing Group, Inc.

6. JRank. (2010). *Battery—Elements*. Available at: http://law.jrank.org/pages/4696/Battery-Elements.html. Accessed June 29, 2010.

7. Medi-Smart. (2010). *Nursing legal issues: How to Protect Yourself*. Available at: http://www.medi-smart.com/nursing-articles/nursing-law/legal-issues. Accessed August 16, 2010.

8. Showers, J. L. (2000). What you need to know about negligence lawsuits. *Nursing, 30*(2), 45–49.

Chapter 14

Labor Laws: Encounters with Unions

Reid M. Oetjen, PhD, *Assistant Professor, Graduate Program Director, e-MSHSA, Department of Health Management and Informatics, College of Health & Public Affairs, University of Central Florida, Orlando, Florida*

Dawn M. Oetjen, PhD, *Associate Professor, Graduate Program Director Health Services Administration, Department of Health Management and Informatics, College of Health & Public Affairs, University of Central Florida, Orlando, Florida*

Chapter Objectives

- Review the current state of labor organizing in the healthcare industry.
- Provide an overview of the history, development, and present state of legislation governing union organizing and operation, including the specific effects on health care of the National Labor Relations Act (NLRA) Amendments of 1974.
- Provide an overview of the collective bargaining process.
- Review the union organizing process, including examination of the reasons why employees organize.
- Review counterorganizing strategies available to employers and describe the role of the first-line manager in addressing union organizing.
- Offer some fundamental advice for first-line managers to consider in ongoing relationships with a union.

Introduction

The healthcare industry is not heavily unionized. In fact, only 10% of total employees in all healthcare settings were members of unions or covered by union contracts in 2006, substantially less than the 13% for all other industries.[1] Additionally, the American Hospital Association reported in 2008 that 27% of the nation's hospitals had some unionized employees.[2] Despite these statistics, the trend in unionization is on the rise. One reason that unions have targeted the healthcare industry is its size; it is second in size only to the federal government, which is already highly unionized. Another reason for targeting health care is found in the unsettled state of the industry; mergers, acquisitions, and other affiliations have led to layoffs in some parts of the system and created uncertainties about job security in what was once referred to as a recession-proof industry.

The number of union petitions for elections in 2009 was on pace to exceed the number in 2008. In 2008, unions held 299 elections and won an overwhelming 72% of them. During the first half of 2009, unions were successful in 113 of 155 elections, or 73% of the time. The number of union organizing attempts for early 2009 already exceeded 155 because unions themselves often call off elections if they feel they cannot win.[3]

In addition to gaining strength in health care, unions have started to work together to push national legislative agenda. Since 2008, three healthcare unions have joined together to create a "super union" to support a new legislative agenda. These efforts include support of card-check legislation, or the Employee Free Choice Act, which proposes to allow the establishment of a union if the majority of employees sign a petition or authorization card, thus bypassing the secret ballot. Union opponents feel that the potential peer pressure, harassment, and coercion that can accompany an open petition may enable unions to quickly make greater headway into the healthcare industry—an industry that in the past shunned the idea of unionization because healthcare workers are typically "called to serve" and are likely to put their interests behind those of their patients. Unions are also working together to support healthcare reform to constrain insurance costs that they feel have prevented them from securing money from employers for wage increases.[3]

Together, these trends in unionization should be a cause for concern for healthcare organizations and managers. This chapter provides an overview of union legislation, a review of several terms and processes involved in unionization, and a discussion of the managerial implications for managing in a union environment. Recommendations are also provided for managers who are either managing employees in the process of unionization or who are managing in a union shop.

An Overview of Union Law

Prior to discussing managerial tactics for dealing with potential unionization or managing in a union environment, a brief discussion of labor law as it pertains to health care is necessary. Because state labor laws vary from state to state, healthcare organizations and their managers need to familiarize themselves with their state and local laws to ensure legal compliance. Many states have separate public employee legislation governing labor agreements and the right to organize, join labor unions, and bargain collectively.[4] This is especially important for state-operated healthcare organizations that are exempt from the National Labor Relations Act (NLRA) and must instead follow state laws.

The National Labor Relations Act of 1935

The critical piece of legislation that changed the landscape of labor law was the NLRA, sometimes referred to as the Wagner Act, enacted in 1935. The NLRA was passed during the period of severe economic turmoil otherwise known as the Great Depression and was an attempt to help get the economy back on track. It marked a significant departure from government policy toward labor organizations; for the first time, workers had the legal authority to be recognized and to bargain collectively.

The NLRA encouraged the rationalization of commerce and industry by establishing minimum wages and maximum hours of work.[5] It also established the National Labor Relations Board (NLRB), which was given the power to investigate charges of unfair labor practices and to conduct elections in which workers would have the opportunity to choose union representation. The NLRB was also given power to facilitate better training and the development of standard procedures in different work areas.[6]

The NLRA gave workers and unions more extensive powers than previous attempts to regulate employee–employer relations had done. The overarching purpose of the NLRA as it pertained to unfair labor practices included the following five limitations on employers.

1. It shall be an unfair labor practice for an employer to interfere with, restrain, or coerce employees in the exercise of the rights guaranteed to workers. . . These rights include the right to self-organize, form, join, or assist labor organizations, to bargain collectively through representatives of their own choosing, and to engage in other concerted activities for the purpose of collective bargaining or other mutual aid or protection. Also, employees have the right to refrain from any or all such activities except to the extent that such right may be affected by an agreement requiring membership in a labor organization as a condition of employment.

2. The Act prohibits employers from dominating or interfering with the formation or administration of any labor organization or contributing financial or other support to it.

3. The Act prohibits discrimination in regard to the hiring process, tenure of employment, or any term or condition of employment that encourages or discourages membership in a labor organization.

4. The NLRA prohibits employers from discharging or otherwise discriminating against an employee for filing charges or giving testimony under this Act.

5. The Act prohibits employers' refusal to bargain collectively with the representatives of their employees. . .[7]

The Taft-Hartley Act (1947)

The Taft-Hartley Act was enacted as a result of growing public discontent toward unions. The Taft-Hartley Act amended the NLRA in four ways: (1) it prohibited unfair union practices; (2) it defined the rights of employees as union members; (3) it defined the rights of employers; and (4) it provided the President of the United States with the power to temporarily bar strikes for reasons of national security, health, and safety.[8]

The Taft-Hartley Act protected employees' rights from the unions and opened the way for right-to-work laws that outlawed labor contracts requiring union membership as a condition of employment. Employers were granted the right to express their views about unions; however, threats, promises, coercion, and direct interference with workers who are trying to reach a decision of whether or not to unionize cannot be used.[8]

The Landrum-Griffin Act (1959)

The 1950s saw further legislation amending the NLRA owing to unethical conduct on the part of some labor unions. The intent of the Landrum-Griffin Act, or the Labor Management Reporting and Disclosure Act, was to protect union members from wrongdoing by their unions. This amendment provided a bill of rights for union members that allowed them to sue their union, and it ensured that no member could be fined or suspended without due process. New protections regarding union elections were also adopted.

The 1974 Amendments to the NLRA

The NLRA did not provide protection for healthcare workers; however, this circumstance changed when the Health Care Amendments to the NLRA were adopted in 1974. These amendments provided labor organizations the right to strike, picket, and engage in other concerted refusals to work at healthcare organizations. The definition of a healthcare institution or organization, according to the NLRA, includes any hospital, convalescent hospital, health maintenance organization, health clinic, nursing home, extended care facility, or other institution devoted to the care of sick, infirm, or aged persons.[7]

Because of the serious nature of health care and the deleterious impact a health-care worker strike could have on the health and safety of patients, several protections were added and are outlined in Section 8(g) of the NLRA as amended in 1974. Specifically, these protections require that all labor organizations provide healthcare organizations a minimum of 10 days notice "before engaging in any strike, picketing, or other concerted refusal to work at any healthcare institution." The intent of this amendment is to provide the healthcare organization with sufficient time to make plans to ensure the continuity of care for patients in the event of a work stoppage.[9]

In the event of a planned strike or other work stoppage, labor organizations are required to notify the Federal Mediation and Conciliation Service (FMCS) of their intention to strike within 30 days after notification of either party's intention to terminate a contract. This, however, does not apply to bargaining for an initial agreement following certification. The FMCS will then appoint an impartial board of inquiry to investigate the issues involved in the dispute and to make a written report to the parties within 15 days after the establishment of a board. The written report includes the finding of fact along with the board's recommendations for settling the dispute, with the objective of achieving a prompt, peaceful, and just settlement of the dispute.

In the event of a work stoppage, healthcare employers have the right to remain open and operational. As such, employers may hire replacement workers to ensure the continuity of care. If the strike is deemed to be an economic strike, in which the workers are attempting to persuade the employer to accept certain terms and conditions of employment, including wage and benefit changes, the healthcare employer has the right to hire "permanent" replacements. However, any striker who is "permanently" replaced must be kept on a preferential hiring list and offered a comparable position if and when one becomes available. An exception to this rule applies if the strike is called in response to an unfair labor practice committed by the employer; when such an event occurs, only temporary replacements can be utilized.[10]

Healthcare employers also have the right to deny or delay the reinstatement of striking workers provided they have legitimate and nondiscriminatory business reasons for doing so. Legitimate business reasons include hiring permanent replacements and entering into temporary staffing contracts. Reinstatement may be difficult for strikers as they may be recalled to a different shift or work unit than their prestrike employment. Thus, a striking worker is not guaranteed to get the exact same job back immediately.

Healthcare employers are also permitted to reasonably restrict union activity in specified areas and times in order to avoid interference with operations. Healthcare employers can also prohibit union activities during employee work hours if such activity is deemed detrimental to patient care and safety.[4]

An additional protection for employers resides in their right to restrict all personal use of the organization's business communication systems by employees. Employers, however, can permit certain types of solicitation at their own discretion. Under this protection, employers can permit solicitations through their communications systems while prohibiting organizational or similar solicitations by employees and employee groups.[11]

Finally, the 1974 amendments allow employers to prohibit their supervisors from participating in union activities. The NLRA defines a supervisor as

> any individual having authority, in the interest of the employer, to hire, transfer, suspend, lay off, recall, promote, discharge, assign, reward, or discipline other employees, or responsibly to direct them, or to adjust their grievances, or effectively to recommend such action, if in connection with the foregoing the exercise of such authority is not merely a routine or clerical nature, but requires the use of independent judgment.[7]

Since this 1974 legislation, several more provisions and amendments have been added.

The Union Election Process

A brief overview of the election process is necessary for understanding how employers can participate and respond during this period. There are five basic steps in the union organizing process.

Initial Contact

The first step of the election process is the initial contact, in which the union assesses the employees' potential interest in organizing. This contact can be initiated either by a union or the employees and usually involves the creation of an organizing committee of employees. During this step, the union educates the committee and others on the advantages of union membership. Laws allow unions to contact employees as long as they do not endanger the performance or safety of the employees or disrupt their work activities. Thus, the majority of contact takes place after hours, during nonworking periods, and off-site.

Authorization Cards

The second step involves petitioning the NLRB to hold an election by showing that a sizable number of employees (at least 30% of the eligible employees in an appropriate bargaining unit) are interested in organizing by having employees sign authorization cards. During this step, both unions and employers often engage in propaganda to win employees to one side or the other. Management is free to weigh in on the issue of unionization; however, neither side may engage in threats, bribes, or coercive behavior.

Management is legally permitted to inform employees of the implications of signing an authorization card and can freely educate workers who have not yet decided to sign cards. Unions are also able to picket the company provided they meet several conditions: (1) they must file a petition for an election within 30 days after the start of picketing; (2) the organization does not already legally recognize another union; and (3) there was not a valid NLRB election during the previous 12 months.

Hearing

During the hearing step, an employer can choose whether or not to contest recognition of the union. If the employer chooses to contest recognition of the union, a hearing will be held for that purpose and also to possibly contest the scope of the bargaining unit, the employees, or employee groups that will be eligible to vote. If the employer does not choose to contest union recognition or the definition of the bargaining unit, no hearing is required.

When an employer contests a union's right to represent employees, the NLRB gets involved and sends a hearing officer to investigate to ensure that an election is appropriate and to determine the scope of the bargaining unit. The bargaining unit is the group of employees who will be represented and bargained for collectively. If deemed appropriate, a hearing will be held to determine if an election should be held.

Campaign

Just as in a political campaign, both sides will appeal to employees for their votes. Unions will ordinarily promise employees a voice in determining wages and working conditions; employers will cite the cost of union dues and the likelihood of special assessments and the sometimes restrictive conditions set forth in a union contract, while emphasizing benefits enjoyed without union involvement. Often the union will give employees the impression that it will "get more" for them without mentioning—as the employer may point out—that bargaining starts with a clean table. That is, the pay and benefits they enjoyed preunion are essentially gone and must be bargained for from scratch.

Both sides are legally restricted from using threats, bribes, or coercion to sway employees, but the employer's actions are spotlighted more clearly than the union's actions. The manager caught up in a union organizing drive would do well to remember the TIPS rule: The employer cannot threaten, interrogate, promise, or spy (more on this later).

Election

The election is held via secret ballot 30 to 60 days after the NLRB issues its Decision and Direction of Election. The NLRB is responsible for providing ballots and other voting materials, including counting ballots, and for certifying the election. A simple majority of votes cast is necessary to win (not a simple majority of those in the bargaining unit) so the turnout for the election can have a strong influence on the outcome. If the employer engages in unfair practices during the campaign, a "no-union" election result may be reversed.[8]

Collective Bargaining

Collective Bargaining Process

If the union election is successful, the next step of the process is collective bargaining. Collective bargaining is a complex process in which union and management representatives negotiate a written contract that details the working conditions. These working conditions typically include wages, benefits, hours, and other work rules.[12] The result of the collective bargaining process is the collective bargaining agreement (CBA) or contract.

The Collective Bargaining Agreement

The CBA is a legally binding contract that: (1) governs the process of negotiation between representatives of a union and employers; (2) outlines the terms and conditions of employment for employees including such items as wages, hours of work, working conditions, and grievance procedures; and (3) defines the rights and responsibilities of trade unions. The parties often refer to the result of the negotiation as a CBA or, sometimes, as the union contract.

Union Security Contracts and Right-to-Work Laws

Union security contracts are usually part of the CBA and detail the extent to which the unions can compel employees to join the union and how union fees will be collected. When labor unions are established, there are typically two types of union security contracts that are established. The first is the *closed shop contract*, where only members of a particular union may be hired. The second, the *union shop contract,* makes continued employment dependent on union membership after a specified amount of time after hire.[13]

Many states have enacted constitutional provisions, or *right-to-work laws*, that make union security contracts illegal. Currently there are 22 states that have enacted right-to-work laws, prohibiting any agreement between labor unions and employers that require membership or payment of union dues a condition of employment. In these states, the *open shop* union security contracts take their place. An open shop is a place of employment where employees are not required to join or financially support the union as a condition of employment.[13]

One last type of union security contract is the *agency shop*. In the agency shop, employers are free to hire union and nonunion employees alike, and these employees are not compelled to join the union as a condition of employment. However, the nonunion employee is required to pay a fee to cover collective bargaining costs.[13]

Why Do Employees Unionize?

Next up for consideration are strategies and methods used to discourage employees from unionizing. The reasons employee groups choose to unionize are numerous, including better wages and benefits, better working conditions, job security, and a collective voice; however, the desire to unionize can typically be attributed to workers' perceptions of management as unfair. When employees feel they are not valued or respected by the employer, they are more likely to unionize. Labor unions initially established a stronghold in US industry to help workers attain safer working conditions, as occurred for example, in the coal-mining industry. Also, unions were able to procure higher wages and better benefits for their members. Unions also obtain employee support because they promise greater job security and stability for their members.

The current trend in unionization in health care continues to gain momentum. This begs the question: Why? One can simply point to management practices that anger workers and ignore their concerns, such as inconsistent and unfair labor practices, perceptions of discriminatory disciplinary actions, unwise management practices, irregular work assignments, and problems with employee scheduling. Also, high executive compensation frequently causes employees to question an organization's commitment to them.

Management Practices Intended to Avoid Unionization

The cost of unionization for employers is a significant aggregate of tangible and intangible costs. Some estimates of the cost of a unionized operation are 25 to 35% greater than for a nonunionized shop. It is important to note that these figures do not include the cost of increased labor and benefits as a result of a CBA. Employer costs also include increased human resource staff necessary to handle grievances and the legal costs necessitated by increased involvement with regulatory agencies such as those associated with hours and wages. Intangible costs include the impact of reduced morale and creativity resulting from employee anger and frustration by virtue of the collective bargaining process enduring for a year or longer, especially when it does not result in the changes promised by the union.[14]

Ultimately, an organization's productivity and reputation for quality often decline markedly when employees unionize. As such, it behooves employers to make all reasonable and legal attempts to avoid unionization because of the severe potential economic consequences. Some tactics that can help ensure that unions are not an attractive or necessary option for an organization's employees follow.

Lines of Communication

The best method of preventing employees from seeking the protection of unions is to open the lines of communication between management and employees. At a minimum, such programs should include "open-door" policies in which employees feel free to discuss issues and concerns with management, thus helping to avoid misunderstanding and thwarting widespread employee discontent. Other effective models of communication include conducting periodic meetings with employee groups that allow workers to share concerns, or having a system for receiving anonymous employee complaints and a method for managers to publicly address them such as the use of an internal intranet website. Frontline managers need to maintain vigilance and should also be sensitive to the "rumor mill" and promptly respond to rumors by providing employees with facts.

Another effective means of aiding communication is through the use of regular surveys to ascertain how employees feel about the terms and conditions of their employment and what they see as areas of concern. Such surveys provide management with significant insight into how they are perceived. Following such a survey, management should share the results with employees along with management's response and possible changes to address issues identified. To allay any fear of reprisal or retaliation, employees should be reassured of the anonymity of such surveys.

Another method for creating an atmosphere of open communication is to incorporate company policies into an employee handbook or manual so employees understand organizational policies, benefit programs, rules of conduct, and other advantages and conditions of employment. Such handbooks set a positive tone for dealing with new employees, letting them know what is expected of them and what they can expect from managers. Another effective method of preventing potential charges of unfair labor practice by workers is to ensure that the content of the handbook complies with all applicable labor laws.[15]

Continuing efforts to improve and establish effective, open communication will help keep employees informed and will build good will with employees. Being proactive and establishing an organization in which open communication is the norm presents some formidable opposition to unionization. Waiting to open communications lines with employees until a union campaign is introduced will be a clear signal to employees that management is interested only because of the potential union threat.

Ombudsman Program

An ombudsman program is a formal program for airing grievances and handling personnel issues in a fair and impartial manner. An ombudsman is a person who acts as a trusted intermediary between an organization and its employees while representing the broad scope of all constituents' interests. Such programs ensure that employee complaints will be reviewed in an impartial manner, thus decreasing the likelihood that workers will be tempted to turn to unions for relief from what may be perceived as poor labor practices. Such formalized policies and procedures help reinforce employee loyalty to the organization.

Train Supervisors

The first line of defense for an organization lies in training frontline supervisors to deal effectively and consistently with employees. Managers should not wait until unionization efforts are underway to do so, but rather, should be proactive to avoid the turmoil of unionization activities. Managers need to be trained regarding how to answer questions about how the organization feels about unions.

It is helpful to create and publicize an official organizational stance on unionization. Many healthcare organizations have formalized policies concerning unions. A carefully crafted statement of the organization's stance, in addition to the rationale for this stance, is critical in helping frontline management communicate the organization's position to employees. Although there are many rules governing how an employer must interact with unions, employers nevertheless have the legal right to oppose unionization and express their opposition to such efforts in a noncoercive manner. Healthcare organizations should consider sharing the union stance with new employees during the orientation process.[15]

Maintain Employee Morale

A potentially effective morale strategy involves motivating employees by implementing formal reward and recognition programs. An effective method often used in developing such programs is to invite employees to offer their ideas concerning motivational practices and ask them what rewards they would consider to be important. Managers need to show appreciation for all employees by openly celebrating successes.

Benefits of increased morale are reduced turnover, fewer absences, and improved quality of service delivery. Creating programs that focus on improved morale will reduce the likelihood of having to convince employees that a union is not needed.

Strive to Be the Preferred Employer

To avoid union activity, a healthcare organization should strive to be the preferred employer in its area. It is recommended that employers keep wages, benefits, and other working conditions on par with those in the area. A noticeable difference in wages and benefits within the community is an invitation for union organizing efforts. Regular wage and benefit reviews are useful to ensure that the employer remains competitive with similar healthcare organizations in the area in which it operates. Membership in state and national associations can provide healthcare organizations with data on salaries and benefits of healthcare workers.

Fair Management Practices

Another effective method for reducing union activity is taking steps to ensure that management and supervisory personnel avoid all unfair labor practices. First-line managers and supervisors should conduct periodic labor-law training to avoid legal pitfalls. Once a union campaign is underway, it is often too late to provide the necessary training. Legal mistakes that can occur during a union drive can seriously undermine an employer's ability to counter organizing efforts on the part of its workers.[15]

Problems invariably arise for organizations that do not enforce rules uniformly and consistently. An organization that allows different supervisors to enforce rules arbitrarily is open to charges of favoritism, not to mention the likelihood of legal charges of unlawful discrimination. For this reason, periodic audits of disciplinary actions, along with supervisory training, can also help to achieve the goal of uniform enforcement of company policies.[15]

Value Employees

One way to show employees they are valued is to empower and encourage them to take responsibility for their work and to incorporate their input into the work processes. Research also suggests that company-paid training is more highly regarded by employees than the provision of certain other benefits. Investing in training and programs that upgrade the skills and education of employees reassures them of their employability and lets them know they are valued members of the organization. Another way to show employees they are valued is to promote from within the organization whenever possible.

Regular informal communications with employees by managers and supervisors are encouraged. These are not scheduled but are rather impromptu one-on-one discussions with employees held to demonstrate concern for them. These meetings should occur during the natural course of business and need not be restricted to workplace topics. Learning more about an employee as a person as well as a producer shows that the organization cares about and values the individual.

When Union Activity Is Present

Despite the best efforts of managers to be fair and impartial, attempts at unionization are often inevitable. When a union targets the organization, managers need to be proactive in the face of tactics that are aimed at tarnishing the organization's reputation and making employees distrustful of management. For instance, unions may highlight quality concerns through the use of local media outlets, including blogs. Also, union organizers may enlist local community leaders in an attempt to block expansion projects.[17]

Organizations must have preparations in place prior to being faced with unionization campaigns. These plans should involve top-level leaders, public relations personnel, and legal counsel in the development strategies to combat union organizing efforts. The first concern should be to ensure that hospital board members and other key personnel are educated on common union strategies. Also, a plan needs to be developed to communicate the organization's stance to community stakeholders to secure their support. A media blitz, including radio, television, and Internet updates, that creates positive publicity can be key to rallying the support of the community. As previously mentioned, unions are well versed in strategies intended to turn communities against organizations.[18]

Federal, state, and local labor laws restrict what managers are permitted to say and do during a union organization campaign. Thus, healthcare organizations need to educate these critical players of the dos and don'ts. Following is a brief outline of how best to interact with rank-and-file employees.

Dos:

- Do remind employees about benefits that are already in place without having to pay union dues.[16]
- Do inform employees that they will be required to pay union dues.[19]
- Do escort outside union officials off the property if they try to solicit employees.[20]
- Do answer employees' questions about union campaign issues and about the organization's present policies.[20]
- Do assure employees that regardless of union status, the organization cares about the employees and will continue to strive to make it a preferred place of employment.[20]
- Do let employees know that management prefers to work directly with them rather than with a third party to settle any potential disputes.[19]
- Do inform employees of the organization's right to hire replacements should they strike for economic reasons.[19]
- Do explain that union representation cannot protect employees from dismissal for cause.
- Do continue to appropriately discipline or dismiss employees that threaten or coerce co-workers either for or against the union.[20]

Don'ts:

- Don't make promises of new benefits during a union election campaign. Only benefits already in place should be discussed; otherwise, the union may lawfully assert promises of benefits for turning down the union.
- Don't threaten employees with job loss if they pursue unionization.
- Don't make unscheduled changes to work schedules, pay, benefits, or working conditions unless the employer can prove they were initiated prior to the start of union activity.

- Don't attempt to spy on union activity or attend union meetings. Even threats that the employer is spying are prohibited.
- Don't prohibit solicitation; employees have the legal right to solicit coworkers on the job site provided it occurs during nonworking time and it does not interfere with the work being performed.[19]
- Don't interrogate employees regarding union activity as this is considered an unfair labor practice.[20]

Rules Regarding Solicitation

During the unionization process, the union will attempt to solicit employees on the job site. Employees belonging to the union are allowed to solicit coworkers verbally and through the use of literature as long as both employees are on nonworking time. Nonworking time includes periods before and after shifts, as well as during breaks, and meal periods. An employer may have the legal right to ban solicitation in the workplace if it is deemed that such solicitation would disrupt healthcare operations.[15]

Employers are permitted to ask nonemployees soliciting employees and distributing union fliers to leave the premises; however, if an employer has previously allowed nonemployee solicitation of other employees, it may not at a later date prohibit union organizers from soliciting in a similar fashion.[17] For instance, if the organization has previously allowed local colleges to solicit employees to pursue advanced degrees, it cannot prohibit similar activity by nonworker representatives of the union.

The Realities of Managing in a Union Environment

Despite the best efforts of organizations to thwart union efforts, union campaigns are often successful. Also, sometimes managers are hired by organizations that already have unionized work groups. Thus it is critical that managers learn to effectively manage in the union environment.

When managers are faced with the prospect of working in a union environment, their initial thoughts are often negative. Some tend to give up, feeling constrained by the restrictive clauses that often result from years of collective bargaining. Rather than adopting a defeatist approach, however, it is critical for managers to remain positive. Adopting an adversarial style and taking a hard-line stance is inappropriate and will likely cause increased anguish and stress.

The union contract should be viewed as a playbook that details the work rules that both managers and employees must follow. It is really no different from the existing labor laws that are imposed by local, state, and federal legislators; the only true difference is that the management of the organization has agreed to additional rules when it negotiated with representatives of the union. If management is unhappy with the terms of the contract, their only recourse is to provide feedback to the administrators responsible for negotiating the contract in hopes that it can be addressed during the next collective bargaining period.

The key item for the manager to remember is that whatever the union contract does not govern remains at the discretion of the manager. If the collective bargaining contract does not cover a particular work rule or facet of an employee's job, the power rests with the manager. So, regardless of the extent of detail in a contract, there are always loopholes and openings for management interpretation without violating the terms of the contract.

Managing Recalcitrant Workers in the Union Environment

One of the benefits of working within a union environment that management inherits is the use of several new informal supervisors in the form of union shop stewards. Shop stewards are appointed by the union to uphold the rights of the employees and are responsible for representing, but not necessarily defending, the workers. This distinction is critical and it is important that management help the shop steward understand this point.

At the same time, the shop steward is an employee of the organization and thus is often a perfect liaison between management and the union. As such, the prudent manager will work closely with shop stewards and take full advantage of the trust that employees place in them, rather than adopting an adversarial stance. It is easier to persuade people politely by using logical arguments rather than being confrontational.

For instance, whenever a potential problem with a particular employee or group of employees arises, it is often useful for management to first meet with the shop stewards to allow them to have the first opportunity to address and perhaps correct the situation. By virtue of allowing shop stewards to deal with recalcitrant employees and other challenging situations, management is empowering them to solve problems without adopting an adversarial role. As a result, management will be perceived as being fair by both the shop stewards and the employees who have entrusted the stewards to use their judgment a nd abilities to solve problems. Often, shop stewards will have the experience and knowledge to correct situations before they get out of hand, thus making management's job easier.

If a situation persists and management must step in to solve the problem, they must make sure the involved employee has the shop stewards available during disciplinary proceedings. Because management has taken the extra step of including the shop stewards, they will find that the stewards are less likely to blindly defend employees, especially when the employee in question has ignored previous good faith efforts by the stewards to seek a solution. Thus, a disciplinary proceeding is often less confrontational than if management had skipped that crucial step. Managers may also find that the employee or employees involved will also be more cooperative and compliant because of the knowledge that management first attempted to let the union resolve the problem or issue.

Conclusion

The growing trend toward unionization is of great concern for healthcare organizations and individual managers. Therefore, organizations should consider the suggestions outlined in this chapter for maintaining open communication. Regardless of what is said by employees and organizers about tangible items such as pay and benefits, the principal reason why employees choose to unionize is their perception that management is, in some way, unfair. That is, the strongest reasons for employees seeking union protection are largely intangible: perceived unfairness, inconsistency of treatment, lack of respect, fears about job security, and other such concerns that cannot be measured in dollars. For the most part, such conditions did not develop overnight; they are often deep-seated and long-standing and cannot be turned around at will by a quickly mounted communications campaign. These conditions developed over the long term and they are reversed only by positive, long-term change.

The individual first-line manager is the key link between higher management and rank-and-file employees and, as such, is responsible for maintaining a culture of trust and open communication. The immediate supervisor is usually the single member of management with whom the employees as a group have the most contact. That immediate supervisor—the first-line manager—is therefore a source of strong influence on the employees' view of the organization, whether for good or for ill—just as the employees view the first-line manager, so too are they often likely to view the organization overall. The essential element of trust takes time to establish, but it can be lost in an instant. Therefore, managers must be proactive regarding employees' concerns, and top management must be responsive to the concerns of the first-line managers.

Despite the best efforts of many healthcare organizations, employee groups continue to seek the protection of unions. Organizations need to be prepared to resist such attempts. In the event of a union organizing campaign, managers need to be trained in how to communicate with employees to get the organization's position across without violating labor laws. Managers must become a source of factual information regarding unions and must be sufficiently knowledgeable to refute false or exaggerated union statements.[21]

In the event that a union campaign is successful, the affected healthcare managers need to accept the fact that they have, by virtue of contractual requirements, acquired several additional constraints on their freedom to manage. However, rather than adopting an adversarial approach, managers can use union stewards to their advantage with managing difficult employees and addressing other day-to-day employee relations issues. A proper, open-minded approach can help minimize the negative effects of managing in a union environment and will enable the manager to direct and manage employees as if the union were not an issue.

Questions for Review and Discussion

1. Why are first-line managers considered the initial line of defense in efforts to keep an organization union-free?
2. Why would most healthcare organizations be best advised to oppose all union organizing attempts?
3. What, if any, healthcare organizations are exempt from the conditions of the NLRA?
4. Why and how does the current state of affairs in the nation's healthcare system invite unionization?
5. Why do newly certified unions invariably ask for improved wages and benefits if employees' greatest concerns, such as unfairness and lack of respect, do not carry price tags?
6. Why is the introduction of a union into the organization not a cost-neutral occurrence for the employer?
7. Why might some first-line managers be of the opinion that working under a union contract is easier than working without a union's presence?
8. What purpose does a comprehensive employee handbook serve when employees may be interested in unionizing?
9. In a unionized environment, in what ways can shop stewards be helpful to department managers?
10. What is the strongest single implication of the proposed Employee Free Choice Act?

References

1. US Department of Labor. (2008, June). *Career guide to industries, 2008–09 edition.* Available at: http://www.bls.gov/oco/cg/cgs035.htm. Accessed November 28, 2009.
2. American Hospital Association. (2008). *Chart book: Organized labor in hospitals, 2008.* Available at: www.aha.org/aha/content/2008/pdf/LABORcharts-080923-print.pdf. Accessed November 3, 2009.
3. Carlson, J. (2009). *Laboring to unite.* Available at: http://www.modernhealthcare.com/article/20091116/REG/911139998#. Accessed November 21, 2009.
4. Pozgar, G. D. (2007). *Legal aspects of health care administration* (10th ed., pp. 403–421). Sudbury, MA: Jones and Bartlett Publishers.

5. Daniel, C. E. (1980). *The ACLU and the Wagner Act: An inquiry into the Depression-era crisis of American liberalism.* Ithaca, NY: New York State School of Industrial and Labor Relations, Cornell University.

6. Millis, H. A. (1950). *From the Wagner Act to Taft-Hartley: A study of national labor policy and labor relations.* Chicago: University of Chicago Press.

7. National Labor Relations Board. (n.d.). *National Labor Relations Act.* Available at: http://www.nlrb.gov/about_us/overview/national_labor_relations_act.aspx. Accessed June 30, 2010.

8. Dessler, G. (2000). *Human resource management* (8th ed., pp. 516–561*).* Upper Saddle River, NJ: Prentice Hall.

9. Sheppard, I. M. (1975). Health care institution amendments to the National Labor Relations Act: An analysis. *American Journal of Law & Medicine, 1*(1), 41–53.

10. King, G. R. (2002, July). *National Labor Relations Act considerations regarding staffing responses to short duration strikes in the health care industry. Labor activity report.* Available at: http://www.jonesday.com/files/Publication/a24be447-83b9-4d1d-86ea-85a6b6a1c559/Presentation/PublicationAttachment/e1902b12-bc78-469b-92c9-933e5249a65a/NLRA.Consideration-Staffing_7-02.pdf. Accessed June 30, 2010.

11. The Guard Publishing Company d/b/a The Register-Guard *and* Eugene Newspaper Guild, CWA Local 37194. (2007, December 16). Cases 36–CA–8743–1, 36–CA–8849–1, 36–CA–8789–1, and 36–CA–8842–1. Available at: http://www.nlrb.gov/shared_files/Board%20Decisions/351/F35170.htm. Accessed October 11, 2009.

12. Buidens, W. (1981, December). Collective gaining: A bargaining alternative. *Phi Delta Kappan, 63*(4), 244–245.

13. Pynes, J. (2004). *Human resources management for public and nonprofit organizations* (2nd ed.). Hoboken, NJ: John Wiley and Sons.

14. Adams, Nash, Haskell, & Sheridan. (n.d.) *What is the cost of unions?* Available at: http://www.anh.com/Content/The_Cost_of_Unions.asp. Accessed October 11, 2009.

15. Gerson, H. E. (1998, May). Avoiding unionization: Tips for employers—healthcare industry—not-for-profit report. *Nursing Homes, 47*(5), 53.

16. Hoffman, H. L. (1989). Personnel practices can help discourage unionization. *Healthcare Financial Management, 43*(9), 48, 50, 52.

17. Qaddumi, T. (2008, July 4). Health care organizations act now to avoid problems with unions. *Houston Business Journal.* Available at: http://houston.bizjournals.com/houston/stories/2008/07/07/focus5.html. Accessed October 12, 2009.

18. Haugh, R. (2006). The new union strategy: Turning the community against you. *Trustee, 59*(10), 14–18.

19. Schuler, R. S. (1987). *Personnel and human resource management* (pp. 536–571). St. Paul, MN: West Publishing Company.

20. Abdelhak, M., Grostick, S., Hanken, M. A., & Jenkins, E. (1996). *Health information: Management of strategic resource.* Philadelphia, PA: Saunders.

21. Oliver, J. (2008, May 5). Unions view health care as ripe filed. *Triangle Business Journal.* Available at: http://houston.bizjournals.com/triangle/stories/2000/05/08/smallb2.html?q=healthcare%20unionization%20avoid. Accessed October 8, 2009.

Chapter 15

Legal Aspects of Employment Documentation: Beyond Medical Records

Charles R. McConnell, BS, MBA, CM, *Health Care Management and Human Resources Consultant, Ontario, New York*

Chapter Objectives

- Differentiate employment documentation from medical documentation and establish its importance to the organization and to the individual manager.
- Review the various types of employment documentation both formal and informal and describe their places as important elements of the organization's employment documentation system.
- Address the legal implications of employment documentation and describe the role some forms of this documentation can assume in employment-related legal actions.
- Review the organization's obligation to supply certain specified documents upon demand by legal order.
- Briefly review the principal retention guidelines for major elements of employment documentation.
- Address the individual manager's role and responsibilities as concerns employment documentation.

Introduction

Most managers in healthcare organizations are well aware of the critical nature of medical documentation. Malpractice lawsuits and legal actions brought by regulatory agencies have made most elements of the healthcare industry sensitive to the difficulties involving inaccurate, inconsistent, or nonexistent medical documentation. Often, a legal proceeding arising from some aspect of patient care centers around a record entry that does not accurately reflect a corresponding order or that is missing, indecipherable, or in some other way lacking. Similarly, the outcome of a legal proceeding can depend on whether the appropriate consent form was executed and can be produced. Increasing numbers of malpractice actions, along with increasing settlements and damage awards and escalating insurance premiums, have heightened awareness of the need for improved clarity, objectivity, and quality in medical documentation.

The patient record in all its forms, whether inpatient chart, outpatient record, or encounter form, seems to be receiving the attention it deserves. Employment documentation, however, remains in a distant second place with many healthcare managers.

For a number of years, employment documentation, consisting of all records concerning an individual employee's relationship with his or her employer, has been increasing in importance. For most managers working in the delivery of health care, employment documentation should be considered as fully important as medical documentation. Although some managers are also caregivers—and are thus directly involved in creating medical documentation or are responsible for its creation—there are many managers who have no involvement with medical documentation. For example, a nursing unit's head nurse will bear responsibility for both employment documentation and medical documentation, but the housekeeping supervisor, the maintenance manager, the business office manager, and the human resources manager will have considerable employment documentation responsibility but not concerned with medical documentation. Regardless of organizational level, every managerial person working in health care has some responsibility for employment documentation.

The Importance of Employment Documentation

Medical documentation is governed almost completely by law, accreditation standards, and professional review processes. However, employment documentation is governed only partially by law and accreditation standards. Much of what can be described as employment documentation arises from adherence to a sense of good business practice and consideration of possible future needs for certain information. Although there are some recognizable legal requirements governing much of an organization's employment documentation, within health care, this area of documentation is not nearly as completely dictated and monitored from without as is the documentation of patient care.

Although record retention requirements exist in most aspects of employment law, other than mentioning a few specific kinds of documents the law provides only limited guidelines as to what the employer must generate and retain. And little or no guidance is provided regarding certain kinds of documentation problems that are likely to arise from time to time.

Kinds of Employment Documentation

The kinds of employment documentation found in healthcare organizations are formal, informal, and initiating or supporting. Within these three general categories are documents that are thoroughly covered in employment law and documents that are not at all covered in employment law.

Formal Documentation

Formal documentation is documentation that is often necessitated by law or regulatory requirement or other outside standard, or that is created in adherence to accepted business practices. It includes most of the items in employee personnel files and a few employee-related records that may be found in places other than the personnel file, such as separately maintained payroll records or employee health records.

Informal Documentation

Informal documentation is not generally covered by law, regulation, or standard. It may be as truly informal or unstructured as a department manager's anecdotal notes (an area of concern to be addressed later). It also consists of memoranda generated in the course of business operations, and internal reports such as those presenting productivity statistics or reporting on employee activities (e.g., progress reports, status reports).

Initiating or Supporting Documentation

This category consists largely of source documentation used in the creation of other records that might themselves be considered formal or informal. For example, an employee time card is a source document for a payroll record; the time card must be retained a certain length of time under the law and the resulting payroll record must be retained even longer. Another example, this one lying on the informal side of initiating or supporting documentation, is a maintenance work order requesting repair of a heating and cooling unit. The work order will likely be the source document for a portion of a maintenance activity report. But what becomes of the completed work order and the resulting activity report is governed solely by the business practices of the organization or perhaps only of the maintenance department.

All of the foregoing kinds of documentation—formal, informal and initiating, or supporting—are potential sources of problems for the healthcare manager.

Problems Arising from Documentation

Documentation can make considerable trouble for managers when they do not have it or it appears not to exist. Also, it can create considerable difficulty for managers when they do have it, but it is poor, weak, inconsistent, incomplete, or generally lacking in some respect. Documentation can also cause problems for managers when there appears to be too little or too much of it.

Most difficulties that arise concerning employment documentation do not ordinarily come from running afoul of some legal requirement, at least not directly. Rather, most problems with employment documentation occur when managers or their organizations are subject to legal actions, whether in the form of complaints filed with employee advocacy agencies such as the Equal Employment Opportunity Commission (EEOC), the state division of human rights, or individual lawsuits brought up by attorneys on behalf of former or current employees.

Legal Implications of Employment Documentation

Every piece of paper even generated relative to a particular employee has the potential to become the key that turns an employee complaint for or against the organization, and thus, for or against the manager.

There are many possible reasons why some former or current employees take their complaints to attorneys or advocacy agencies. People who feel they have not been heard within the organization will indeed be heard when they sue the employer or complain to an advocacy agency. The employee who sues the employer or otherwise files a complaint is suddenly no longer talking to a deaf ear, if that indeed had been the case. Rather, the individual is now talking with attorneys who have settlement authority and enjoy ready access to upper management or with agency officials who likewise have access to management because they have the force of the law behind them.

Like many other laws, those governing employment relationships are not hard, fast, and inflexible rules. Rather, they are principles and guidelines that are often subject to interpretation. As far as employment law is concerned, much of the time, a wrong is not in fact a wrong but is merely a perception that something wrong has been done or an injustice has been committed.

Employment law and the laws governing individual lawsuits fall under the heading of civil law. There are some significant differences between civil law and criminal law. For an individual or organization to be charged with wrongdoing under criminal law, there must be some legal basis for the charge. There must be some indication that a crime or misdemeanor has been committed, and there must be a demonstrable connection between that act and the individual or organization being charged. There may perhaps be an arrest resulting from a direct connection with the occurrence of an incident, or there will perhaps be an indictment resulting from a grand jury proceeding.

Under civil law, however, there need not be a direct and immediately demonstrable connection with a wrongdoing. There can be no arrest and charge under criminal law based on someone's notion of a perceived wrong that is generally unsubstantiated. However, under civil law it is just that—the notion of a perceived wrong—that ordinarily triggers a legal action. An individual who believes he or she has been wronged by the work organization need only make a statement of sufficient clarity to encourage an advocacy agency to look into the matter or need only secure an attorney who will take on the matter and file a lawsuit.

Thus, a formal complaint pursued by an advocacy agency or a lawsuit brought by an attorney, either of which the organization must defend itself against, can result from an individual's perception of having been done an injustice. A great many employment-related complaints and lawsuits do in fact arise from individual perceptions of wrongdoings. An advocacy agency such as the EEOC will ordinarily pursue most of the complaints it receives; that is why this agency exists. Although such an agency will ordinarily screen out obviously frivolous or clearly unfounded complaints, as long as its representatives agree that there is a chance of actual wrongdoing related to the complainant's perception of wrong, the agency will pursue the matter and the organization that has been charged will have to expend resources responding to the complaint.

An individual can, of course, take his or her grievance to a private attorney who may take on the matter and file a lawsuit.

When work begins in earnest on attempting to resolve a formal complaint or lawsuit, the advocacy agency or the employee's attorney is likely to seek out employment-related documentation of several kinds. An advocacy agency will use much of this documentation in making its decision on the complaint. But it is often extremely difficult to comply with an agency's request for documentation. It is sometimes necessary to furnish literally thousands of pages of paper that must be sifted and sorted from years worth of records and copied. And it is potentially even more difficult to comply with the documentation requests arising in an individual lawsuit.

Not all employment-related lawsuits go all the way to the courtroom. A great many (likely the vast majority) are resolved by settlement at some point along the path to the courtroom. Some lawsuits end along the way by being thrown out by a judge as unworthy, and many are settled out of court. Sometimes management will agree to settlement on the advice of legal counsel because pursuit of the case has revealed management to be vulnerable in some respects. Sometimes the organization, although believing no wrong has been done, will elect to cut its losses rather than face the expense and inconvenience of a protracted legal battle.

A strategy frequently followed by plaintiff's attorneys in employment-related cases involves deliberately making the process so inconvenient, frustrating, confusing, time-consuming, and expensive for the organization that management will be eager to settle. And although settlement usually means that monetary damages paid to the plaintiff are less than those originally sought, it also means that the plaintiff does achieve a victory of sorts and that the plaintiff's attorney gets paid. Negotiated legal fees are usually part of every settlement. And it is within the pursuit of the legal strategy of tying up the organization's time and resources for protracted periods that employment documentation becomes so important.

Documentation thus becomes one of the opposition's major weapons in the legal process known as discovery—that is, the process of seeking out evidence and questioning involved parties in establishing a case. The trigger that brings this weapon into play is the *notice to produce,* a legal notice requiring that certain specified kinds of documentation be furnished. This notice is often served in conjunction with one or more notices of deposition requesting the presence of certain involved parties for questioning by the plaintiff's attorney.

Also touched upon in earlier chapters, the notice to produce is furnished under what is referred to as a federal rule of civil procedure. The notice indicates that under this rule, the organization is "required to produce for copying and inspection" essentially anything that may be thought to be related to the charge in question in any way.

Sometimes the discovery phase may be described as a protracted fishing expedition in which the plaintiff's attorney looks for anything that may eventually be used to support the allegations in the lawsuit. Subject to an often generous time limit, the fishing expedition may range over many grounds for a considerable time. This sometimes leaves participants who are subject to deposition wishing there was some way to end the case so they could get back to the business of running the organization.

It is, of course, possible to file objections to the sometimes seemingly outlandish demands of a notice to produce. However, the objection process can be somewhat cumbersome and time consuming. Ordinarily, the organization defending itself against a particular charge or set of charges will have to furnish a great deal of paper and put up with a great deal of questioning. Consider some examples of documents requested in a notice to produce served in a case involving a former employee who sued an organization for denying an advancement opportunity on the basis of age and sex:

- The personnel file or any personnel document, in whatever form or forms maintained, including, but not limited to performance appraisals, pay records, discipline records, training and experience records, job assignment records, transfer or promotion records, and all other related records for . . . (a list of the names of more than 20 people appeared here);
- The institution's personnel policy manual in all of its forms and revisions as existed at any time during the complainant's employment;
- Copies of any rules, policies, or regulations that the manager alleges the plaintiff violated at any time during his or her employment, or that the manager alleges any other employees of the department broke at any time;
- All writings related to the manager's handling of any alleged violation of rule, policy, or regulation by the plaintiff or by any other employee;
- All job postings, advertisements, or announcements made in any respect, whether internal or external, for any job openings occurring in the department at any time during the plaintiff's employment;

- All writings related to the hiring or transfer into the department of all persons in the department during the plaintiff's employment (the names of nearly 50 present and former employees appeared here); and
- The document or documents that the manager is believed to have on file in the department, including notes maintained by the present manager, in addition to employee files originated by the previous manager, including all comments, whether positive or negative, from the beginning of keeping such notes or records to the present.

Although the foregoing are cited simply as examples, they were adapted from a real case in which these requests were but 7 of more than 40 document requests. Meeting these demands ranged from producing a single slip of note paper to providing file boxes filled with documents.

Again, all of this, which some might be tempted to label legal harassment, is a sometimes necessary part of pursuing a lawsuit. It should be kept in mind, however, that much of this document-request activity may be initiated by the plaintiff's attorney in an effort to create a climate conducive to settlement while pursuing a wide-ranging fishing trip for evidence. Every piece of paper that may be even remotely connected to anything that could lead to pertinent information is susceptible to this process.

The organization is obligated to make all requested information available, but the plaintiff's attorney, and therefore the plaintiff, must bear the cost of copying. In the case from which the above examples were abstracted, the copying loomed as so voluminous that the organization made space available for the plaintiff's attorney to bring in a copier and a clerk to spend several days copying. The organization, as any other organization would be in a similar situation, was within its rights to insist that none of its original documentation be removed from the premises.

It would pay for the manager to always be mindful that every piece of paper generated that even remotely concerns a particular employee is a potential exhibit in a legal proceeding. Of course, much employment documentation lies well beyond the control of the individual manager, including most of what is maintained in an individual's personnel file and how long it is retained. It nevertheless behooves the manager to understand the documentation requirements of the system, even though much of the system's operation lies beyond the manager's control. However, there is much important documentation that the manager can control or greatly influence.

In the area of controllable employment documentation, there are a few things the manager can do during the day's work to ensure that life will be easier than it might otherwise be if the organization is sued under employment law.

Obviously, whatever the documentation system requires and what the manager does overlap in a number of places. For example, the organization's system may require that performance appraisals and written warning notices be used under certain circumstances. But exactly how these are completed is left to the manager. And certainly it is often the manager's responsibility to ensure that such pieces of system documentation find their way into the appropriate personnel files.

To make the best of any opportunities to control employment documentation, it is first necessary to understand the organization's employment documentation system, and then to consider how the manager should work within the system to influence the quality of employment documentation.

The Employment Documentation System

The Personnel File

The manager generally has limited control over what kinds of documents go into the personnel file. As already noted, however, the manager can control whether some items that should go into the personnel file do indeed get there.

Although its contents can vary somewhat, the personnel file will ordinarily include: employment application; résumé, if any; reference checks; employee benefits enrollment forms; employee handbook receipts; personnel actions, such as grade, pay, and title changes and departmental assignment changes; and employee status changes such as a change in marital status or address. Also ordinarily found in the personnel file are performance appraisals, commendations or special notices, disciplinary actions, and verifications of employment and income for credit purposes. Some forms relating to an employee's use of workers' compensation or disability insurance may appear in the personnel file, but the medically related information accompanying these will ordinarily be—or at least should be—held in a separate personnel health file. Such files actually constitute medical records and are thus subject to stricter standards of control.

Concerning the maintenance and confidentiality of personnel records, the organization should have an official policy governing access to them. Only persons who have a legitimate need to know should have access to personnel records. Individuals with a business need to know would ordinarily include:

- Certain employees of the human resources department;
- A particular employee's immediate supervisor and that supervisor's superiors;
- The organization's legal counsel; and
- Interested supervisors and managers who may be considering a particular employee as a transfer candidate.

However, employee privacy is a rapidly growing concern and the access requests by even anyone included in the aforementioned categories should be carefully considered to make certain that a legitimate business need to know exists before a particular personnel file is made available.

The personnel record policy should also control the disclosure of personnel record information to outside agencies and individuals, requiring either written employee consent or legal subpoena or court order for disclosure, and include language clearly intended to protect the confidentiality of such records.

The policy should also include a provision describing the circumstances under which employees may be allowed to view their personnel records. Such review will ordinarily be permitted by appointment and in the presence of a human resources representative. Although an employee will not be permitted to remove anything from the personnel file—even though the file contains confidential information about the employee, it remains the property of the organization. However, the employee may be permitted to enter objections, explanations, or other comments into the record should he or she desire to do so.

Significant problems in employment litigation can be created by gaps in the personnel file. In an organization that may have hundreds or even thousands of personnel files, it is not unusual for occasional performance appraisals, pension statements, disciplinary actions, employee handbook receipts, rate-change notifications, and the like to be missing. When a particular item is not found in the file where it is thought to be, it is a common reaction to wonder whether the item was misplaced, or perhaps wonder if the item does not exist either because it was destroyed or never generated in the first place. A simple but important step the manager can take to ensure that gaps in the personnel file are kept to a minimum is to faithfully send to the human resources department the record copies of all appropriate documents as soon as they are generated.

Another problem commonly encountered in personnel files consists of documents that are not filed in chronological order. In many personnel record systems, documents are filed in the order in which they are received. This is not necessarily the order in which they are generated and dated. Also, when files are unbound so certain documents can be copied, the files are not always reassembled in their original order. Although not nearly as serious as missing documentation, the lack of chronological order can add to the difficulties encountered in locating all documents pertinent to an employment litigation.

The Personnel Health Record

While in some ways it is considered part of the personnel file, an employee's personnel health file is primarily a medical record. As such, it should be maintained separate from the personnel file. Far stricter rules of confidentiality apply to the personnel health record. As with medical records in general, information from the personnel health record moves from and to medical personnel legitimately involved in the medical care of the individual and then only with the consent of the individual (who in this instance is more properly identified as a patient than as an employee). Personnel health records maintained in the personnel file, as once was commonly the case in many organizations, are subject to casual scrutiny by far more persons than have a legitimate medical or legal reason to know. Also, the availability of this information can lead to other problems. Consider, for example, the case of an employee who successfully pursued a claim that he was denied a transfer opportunity because of an occasionally recurring medical condition that caused the manager to decide he was an attendance risk.

Personnel Record Retention

A document that no longer exists cannot be called upon in a legal action, and there are indeed some documents that can be destroyed after a specified amount of time. However, the legal guidelines for personnel record retention are a grand mixture of sometimes conflicting and frequently overlapping requirements. Because of the maze of regulations involved, it is becoming increasingly more risky to destroy any employment documentation.

In addition to a variety of state laws, there are federal requirements governing most employment documentation. Within the federal laws, for example, one will find that:

- Under the Fair Labor Standards Act (FLSA), records concerned with wages, hours, and conditions of employment must be retained for at least 3 years.
- Records designated in the Equal Pay Act must be retained for 3 years.
- Under the Age Discrimination in Employment Act (ADEA), certain information must be retained for at least 1 year, whereas other documents must be kept for at least 3 years.
- The Employee Retirement Income Security Act (ERISA) requires that certain key documents be retained for at least 6 years.
- The Occupational and Safety Health Administration (OSHA) calls for some documents to be retained for as long as 20 years; subsequent legislation such as New York state's Right-to-Know Law, dealing with exposure to toxic substances, requires that certain documents be retained for as long as 40 years.

The threshold for retaining most employment documentation is 6 years. Because 6 years also happens to be the statutory limit for filing most employment-related actions, one might conclude that a personnel file could be destroyed in its entirety 6 years after a particular employee leaves the organization. However, there are still the OSHA and other longer-term requirements to consider. There are also legitimate references checks and other requests that regularly call for access to records that are older than 6 years. Today, it is perhaps more appropriate to retain personnel files indefinitely, although certain records that are more than 5 or 6 years old can be committed to microfilm for ease of storage while remaining available for information they may contain.

Other Employment Documentation System Elements

The organization's performance appraisal form is part of the formal documentation system. Also belonging to the system are warning, suspension, and discharge notices and all other paperwork related to disciplinary actions. Employee transfer requests may also be part of the system. And although they do not ordinarily appear in personnel files, job descriptions are part of the formal employment documentation system.

If any of the foregoing or other items that have not been mentioned are generated because they are organizational requirements, they become part of the documentation system and most will find their way into personnel files.

Paper Volume

One piece of paper does not seem like much. Two, three, or four pieces of paper do not seem like much. However, when everything generated concerning employment is considered, it amounts to a significant volume of paper. Paper volume should be kept in mind by all who design forms and paperwork systems or who use or contribute to these processes. It is always wise to think twice before creating a new form if an existing form can be revised to do the work of two or if a two-part form could realistically replace a three-part form.

Simply put, the more paperwork there is, the more difficult it becomes to keep track of it all. When an organization is involved in employment litigation, the more paper there is, the more paper can be called forth via a notice to produce, and the more difficult it becomes to locate any single document.

Today, a considerable amount of employment-related information that exists on paper also exists in electronic form. However, for most organizations, the personnel file in its entirety remains in hard copy.

The Manager and Employment Documentation

Coping with employment documentation requires a conscientious attitude toward paperwork and a determination to keep the essential documents timely, accurate, and complete. Some managers tend to shy away from paperwork; however, they need to accept this work as essential to doing a complete job and determine to stay on top of it as much as possible.

Maintain Anecdotal Note Files

It is helpful for the manager to keep anecdotal note files, preferably a separate file for each employee. These files will ordinarily contain miscellaneous information that is not sent to the central personnel files, including notes on discussions held or problems encountered, or notes both positive and negative relating to employee performance that will eventually be reflected in an employee's next performance appraisal. This anecdotal note file may also hold records of disciplinary actions that do not go into the central personnel file, such as the circumstances surrounding oral warnings or counseling sessions.

The anecdotal note file will generally contain informally recorded information pertinent only to the manager and the individual employee (i.e., information that does not go into the individual's personnel file). However, the anecdotal file may also include the manager's copies of the employee's performance appraisals and other personnel documents such as warning notices that have already been placed in the official personnel file.

Not everything the manager needs or wishes to retain relative to his or her relationship with a particular employee must, or even should, ever find a permanent home in the official personnel file. Much of this informal documentation, which may be temporary and pertinent to a particular manager and employee relationship, should be kept in the anecdotal file.

Follow All Applicable Procedures

The manager should never give in to the temptation to take shortcuts by skipping or skimping in creating the formal documentation required by the organization's system. If a document must be initiated or a form generated, this should be accomplished in timely fashion providing all required information—including dates and signatures, elements that are often critical in employment litigation.

Concerning records of disciplinary actions, the manager should also endeavor to obtain employee signatures. An employee who is subject to disciplinary action should be reminded that he or she has the right—and is indeed encouraged—to note comments or objections on the pertinent document. However, an employee may occasionally refuse to sign a warning under any circumstances; when this occurs, the manager should note the employee's refusal to sign and, if possible, have the refusal witnessed by another manager. Many employees who refused to sign a warning have later claimed to have never seen the document.

Concerning performance appraisals, each appraisal conference should be accomplished in a timely fashion with the organization's appraisal form completed in full and signed by the employee. The employee should be encouraged to enter comments or objections and be advised that signing is not meant to indicate agreement with the appraisal but rather to simply acknowledge that it has been received and discussed. Honest, realistic appraisals are potentially quite important in certain employment-related lawsuits. When an employee is terminated for performance issues, there had best be recent appraisals on file reflecting performance problems. If an employee so terminated can point to a satisfactory rating on an appraisal hastily concluded by a manager who would just as soon quickly get out from under the task, it can be used to refute the termination.

Job descriptions, another common element of formal employment documentation, are rarely complete and up-to-date at all times. Yet incomplete or outdated job descriptions can cause problems related to job content. An employee's seemingly insubordinate refusal to perform a task that "Isn't in my job description" can, under certain circumstances (think unionized employees) be upheld. It falls to the manager to make every reasonable effort to maintain current job descriptions.

Other documents, such as transfer requests, also require careful and consistent handling. Many transfer request forms require the manager to provide a statement explaining why the particular transfer candidate was not accepted. Much candidate assessment consists of a manager's gut feelings as well as a review of qualifications. Gut feelings, however, cannot be objectively documented, and a manager is sometimes led to fabricate a rejection based on experience and qualifications that might not stand up when compared with the experience and qualification of other candidates.

Dates Are Important

As noted earlier, dates can be especially important with employment documentation. Missing dates are ordinarily not prevalent in the formal documentation that enters the official personnel file, but they often abound in informal documentation such as anecdotal notes and handwritten statements and accounts of various events. In many employment-related cases, difficulties have arisen and controversies created because nobody was able to say with certainty when a particular document was generated.

There is a simple but important rule that every manager should faithfully observe: Never set pen or pencil to paper without first dating the page.

Use Accurate, Objective Language

Subjective assessments, emotional language, inflammatory terminology and name-calling should be kept completely out of informal documentation. This admonition should apply in even the most personal of documentation that a manager believes no other person will ever see (i.e., no terms such as lazy, uncooperative, arrogant, argumentative, unmotivated, gossipy, etc.). As a general rule, the manager should use only language that appears in the organization's work rules and disciplinary procedures when describing an employee's behavior, whether suspected or proven.

The ideal approach to language use embodies a manager's determination to put nothing on paper that might cause embarrassment or discomfort if it went public. When files are brought into the legal process, they are indeed public, in that they are opened to far more eyes than those of the manager who created them. If the files include emotional, inflammatory, or slanderous remarks or labels or if they contain outlandish charges that cannot be substantiated, the opposition's legal counsel can make life difficult for the manager.

Check for Errors

Many people perform a great many business tasks on a once-through basis, completing forms or generating other documents without checking what has been done.

This tendency is especially apparent in informal documentation when thought and observations are simply jotted down. Also, many people are even more inclined to go once-over-lightly when working under time constraints. There are bound to be documentation errors from time to time, but the manager can minimize these by proofreading each document or note before filing it or sending it on its way.

In employment litigation, simple errors made in all innocence can become extremely troublesome. For example, in one particular case, an employee claimed that he was a Technician II, a grade 5 in the salary system, when in fact he had been designated and paid as a Technician I, salary grade 4. Claiming that since a Technician II was paid at a higher rate but that he had been receiving Technician I pay for several years, he produced a job description that identified his position as Technician II and three performance appraisals on which his position was entered as Technician II. Investigation revealed that an early titling error on the initial job description began a chain of events that spread the erroneous title and grade throughout the employer's system, a single error ultimately emerging in the form of trouble.

Someone, in all probability a plaintiff's attorney, will use lax recordkeeping and errors or gaps in employment documentation to create doubt. Where there is room for doubt, there is room to instill the belief that something done in error might actually have been done willingly or maliciously.

Periodically Clean Out the Files

If anything exists in writing, even in so-called personal files, it can be accessed by opposing legal counsel. That is, *if* it exists.

Aside from matters of producing documents for litigation, it is simply good business to periodically rid files of excess baggage. The manager should critically view boxes of aging documentation (such as old work-order slips) that take up space but are not subject to legal retention requirements. Most such material will never be accessed again for business need, but when it is requested by an attorney attempting to build a case, it can suddenly present problems of sheer bulk.

However, it is necessary to purge aging documentation, and especially anecdotal notes, before this material is demanded in a legal notice to produce. The phrasing appearing in a notice to produce may include: "Notes in whatsoever form on (employee's name)" or "Any writings in whatsoever form concerned with . . ." The manager may see in the legal notice that an anecdotal note file is thought to exists on "information and belief." This is the opposition's way of saying, "We have reason to believe such a file exists, so if it does exist we want it."

Important to remember: It is all right to purge files in the normal course of business, but this cannot be done once a notice to produce arrives. Once the notice is in hand, it becomes a violation of law to destroy any requested documentation even though the persons who served the notice may not be absolutely certain that the records really exist.

Other factors should be considered when handling most formal documentation and probably a great deal of informal documentation. According to a policy implemented by the EEOC in 1986, the destruction of personnel records by employers facing investigation by the EEOC may be used as evidence that illegal discrimination has occurred. The EEOC may then find discrimination based on an investigation that is less than complete when an employer withholds records from investigators. If records are missing, the EEOC will take steps to determine why a respondent to a discrimination charge did not keep the records as required by regulations. If it is found that a respondent knowingly destroyed or knowingly failed to keep certain records in anticipation of a charge of discrimination, investigators can draw what is referred to as an *adverse inference* that the missing information would have been unfavorable to the respondent.

Good Business

Good documentation is good business. Good documentation is also one of the manager's best defenses in employment litigation.

Legal considerations aside, it is easier to operate effectively when all available documents say what they ought to say and are found where they ought to be found, and when those documents that have outlived their practical and legal usefulness have been destroyed.

On the legal side of the documentation discussion, one primary tactic for wearing management down toward settlement is seemingly endless discovery and continual chasing of documents in response to one or more notices to produce, all of which can continue until the assigned judge calls it to a halt.

A manager must control documentation and never let documentation itself take control. Complete, honest, and objective documentation, every piece created as though it might go public or be subject to legal scrutiny, will work *for* the manager far more often than it can be forced to work *against* the manager.

Questions for Review and Discussion

1. If the majority of important documents in a personnel file are subject to specific, known retention periods, why is it suggested that personnel files are best retained indefinitely?

2. Why might the organization willingly settle a lawsuit in spite of management's belief that no wrong was committed?

3. Why is it necessary to keep health-related documentation such as workers' compensation and disability records separate from an individual's personnel file?

4. Describe the problems that can result when undated documentation finds its way into a legal proceeding.

5. In what ways can a manager's personal anecdotal note files exert a negative influence in a legal proceeding?

6. Describe several reasons why an aggrieved employee would take his or her complaint to an attorney or an outside advocacy agency.

7. How can giving an underperforming employee a satisfactory performance appraisal rating backfire on a manager?

8. Describe the problems to be encountered in a legal proceeding because of incomplete or nonexistent documentation.

9. If one employee has initiated a lawsuit, why might the employee's attorney demand copies of the personnel files of everyone in the department?

10. Offer at least two significant reasons why a plaintiff's attorney might insist, via the notice to produce, on access to extensive files and records.